BE STRONG AND SURRENDER

A 30 DAY RECOVERY GUIDE

Pastor Philip Dvorak
Dr. Paul Meier
Dr. Jared Pingleton

Be Strong and Surrender
A 30 Day Recovery Guide

Published by Recovery Resources
Printed by Pen Culture Solutions   11/26/2022

Pen Culture Solutions
1-888-727-7204 (USA)
1-800-950-458 (Australia)
support@penculturesolutions.com

ENDORSEMENTS

Anyone who delves into their own spiritual growth must ultimately come face to face with their own brokenness, sin, and hurt. Healing and recovery are some of the deepest aspects of what it means to be a person of faith, and of what the Bible teaches us. The authors provided a resource that you will want to keep on your bedside, as you have your devotional times. You will read scripturally based principles and stories that will encourage and help you to surrender your life in God's strength, and ultimately to be transformed. Highly recommended!

John Townsend, Ph.D., *New York Times* bestselling author of more than 30 books selling over 10 million copies, Leadership Consultant, and Licensed Clinical Psychologist

As a founder of a treatment center and being in this field over 35 years, it's rare that a new resource comes along that is a *must have*. The carefully crafted words in this book give hope and will empower you to walk strong in your recovery. This is a healing and hope filled book that we use at *The Center A Place of HOPE* (in Edmunds, WA).

Gregory L. Jantz, Ph.D., Founder, The Center A Place of HOPE, bestselling author of over 40 books, Edmunds, WA

Clear, well-written, and compelling, *Be Strong and Surrender* will aid your healing journey by feeding your mind with scriptural truth and leading your soul closer to Jesus, the Healing One.

John Stumbo, D.Min., President, The Christian and Missionary Alliance and author of several books.

Practically everyone I know has a family member or friend that has been deeply damaged by the 'idolatry of addiction.' The solution to our present catastrophe—and all others—is Jesus. To quote one of the authors, "Jesus is not a higher power. He is the highest power."

Countless lives have been drastically transformed by the power of His Name, and I believe many more will be changed as a result of reading *Be Strong and Surrender*. There are a lot of good books out there, but none more needed than this one, for it points each of us to The One, The Only One who can set us free. Forever!

David Nelms, D.Min., Founder and President, The Timothy Initiative

Spirituality and faith are the foundations of sobriety and recovery. *Be Strong and Surrender* opens us to receive God and fully experience the joys of recovery.

Bill Russell, former CEO, The Treatment Center of the Palm Beaches, Palm Beach, FL

As an owner and hands-on manager of an addiction treatment center, I have watched, cheered, suffered, and mourned the lives of many clients. When I was approached to review this book, I welcomed a new way to see the light of a truly higher power. I was pleased to read the honest and easy-to-grasp concept of their approach to recovery. I strongly encourage the addicted, their families, and friends to participate in reading this book. Too often authors try to impress readers with their knowledge, which usually leaves us wondering what they meant. Now we are offered a humble explanation with a compete referenced guide. Please enjoy the journey and then share it with friends and family members.

Mark Gerhardt, President, Transformations Treatment Center, Delray Beach, FL

Small changes in trajectory lead to dramatic shifts in direction over time. Those who choose to shift their direction from addiction to recovery through surrender to Jesus undertake a noble endeavor indeed. Be Strong and Surrender will be an invaluable resource for any and all setting out on that path. I would know – I'm 18 years sober from intravenous drug addiction, homelessness, psychiatric care, and despair! The words in the pages to follow map the path from that kind of brokenness into a life of true peace, gratitude, and joy.

Trent Langhofer, Ph.D., Professor at Colorado Christian University, former pastor at Whites Ferry Road Church, Monroe, LA (known as the "Duck Dynasty" Church), Licensed Professional Counselor

It has been said that addiction is the biggest public health crisis of our time. Spreading the message of recovery needs to be on the agenda of every leader. *Be Strong and Surrender* is an opportune, practical, and insightful resource that should be in the hands of every person in recovery and every servant leader that supports them.

James Davis, D.D., President, World Leaders Group

These authors display a unique blend of multidisciplinary expertise which skillfully leads the reader into a deep heart reflection and examination while equipping them with practical life tips for not only enhanced recovery success, but for life transformation.

Karl Benzio, M.D., Co-founder and Medical Director, Honey Lake Clinic, Greenville, FL, founder and Director, Lighthouse Network

DEDICATION

This book is dedicated to all those who have been impacted by the destructive and deadly struggles of alcoholism and substance abuse. This is to those who are currently suffering, to those who have felt like they have lost the fight, and to those who have lost those they love. May this book inspire you to find help, healing, and hope.

CONTENTS

ACKNOWLEDGMENTS

To all those who have sacrificed to make this resource a reality:

Our wives, children, family, and friends who put up with our eccentricities and at times inaccessibility in order to allow us to complete this important work. We love you and thank you for loving us. You are simply the best!

Bill Russell – A true man of peace.

Nancy Brown – A true servant leader.

Patty Roberts – The best eagle eye we know.

FOREWORD

We face an enormous and unprecedented crisis today in our country, our churches, and our homes. Alcohol and opioid addictions are raging out of control and are getting worse every day. Many are calling the scourge of addiction the number one social, mental, relational, spiritual, and public health problem in our society.

Be Strong and Surrender is a most timely and inspirational recovery resource. This unique, easy to read, 30-day recovery devotional study guide should be in the hands of every person in recovery as well as those who love and help them. Pastors, support group leaders, professional clinicians, and all people who come alongside persons struggling with addictions will find rich insights to find comfort, help, hope, and victory. Drawing from the authors' over nine decades of combined professional experience ministering to hurting persons, this daily devotional study is filled with powerful and profound biblical and psychological truths which will encourage, equip, and empower people to face their addictions with courage and confidence.

These three men are the perfect combination of integrity, experience, and insight. Pastor Phil Dvorak is fast becoming one of the foremost leaders in the field of Christian addiction treatment. His compassionate, insightful, yet firm approach connects to your heart in a truly life giving way. Dr. Paul Meier is considered by many as a founding father of the Christian psychology movement and in *Be Strong and Surrender* provides the reader with remarkable insights that can be easily applied to a person's journey of recovery. Dr. Jared Pingleton is a clinical psychologist, dedicated minister, and acclaimed author who is a respected national leader in the Christian mental health field. He superbly integrates a solid biblical and clinically sound perspective into practical thought-provoking tools for the recovery journey.

Tim Clinton, Ed.D., President, American Association of Christian Counselors, Co-host of Family Talk Radio, and author of over 30 books.

DAY ONE

Word of the Day: *Surrender*

Scripture: "If you try to hang on to your life, you will lose it. But if you give up your life for my sake, you will save it. And what do you benefit if you gain the whole world but lose your own soul? Is anything worth more than your soul?" (Matthew 16:25-26, NLT)

Quote: "Some of us have tried to hold on to our old ideas and the result was nil until we let go absolutely." (Alcoholics Anonymous, 1st. Edition)

Say Uncle

I'm the youngest child of four (Phil). I have two older brothers and an older sister. I know a little about surrendering. As a child I always seemed to be the one running behind, trying to catch up... My brother Matt would wrestle me to the ground on a regular basis. I guess he loved watching "professional wrestling." I was the one he practiced his newest wrestling moves on. Matt was four years older. It really wasn't fair. Needless to say, he would always win. I remember being pinned down on multiple occasions with my brother yelling "say uncle." Finally, after what felt like a lifetime I would give in, feeling defeated, bruised and humiliated.

A part of me hates the word surrender. It brings words to my head, like "say uncle." I feel like a coward, a wimp, a failure, a loser, etc. I feel like something just died inside me. But what's so funny about this is that it couldn't be further from the truth.

1

Surrender is about life. People surrender because they want to live; almost no one surrenders to die. Surrender is about living. When we surrender, paradoxically we can begin to truly live. Humor me for a second as I share a lesson I learned from Pastor Craig Groeschel. Put your hands up. Yes, put your hands up in the air. What is this a symbol of? Yes it's a universal symbol of surrender. Now imagine you're at your favorite sports game. Put your hands up in the air. It's now a symbol of victory. The same action is both the universal symbol of surrender and victory. Surrender is often our only true path to victory.

Jesus said "If you try to hang on to your life, you will lose it. But if you give up your life for my sake, you will save it. And what do you benefit if you gain the whole world but lose your own soul? Is anything worth more than your soul?" Matthew 16:25-26 (NLT)

I've spent the majority of my life searching, longing, desiring to be happy, to be fulfilled. I tried to save myself for years. I tried to hang on to living life on my own terms. I would give God a little, but still try to hang on to something. It always worked out the same way--it didn't matter if it was alcohol, sex, porn, money, whatever I tried to fill that void with, the more I hung on, the more I lost. My efforts were futile and ineffective.

Sometimes in life we are so busy carrying around our junk that we can't pick up the gifts that God is trying to give us. "If you try to hang on to your life, you will lose it." If you try to hang on to parts of your old life you will lose your new life. Jesus doesn't mince words here. You cannot hold on to parts of your old life and live a new life. It doesn't work that way. If you want to live a life of sobriety, a new life, a healthy life, if you want your family, your marriage, your friendships restored, whatever the brokenness, you must surrender it all to Jesus.

This seemingly contradictory principle is actually a profound and prime example of how the mysterious Kingdom of heaven functions. Jesus frequently taught eternal concepts of God's wise and mature way of living by using what my (Jared's) favorite professor in graduate school called the "Mystery of the Inverse Order."

Throughout the Gospels, Jesus would use humanly unconventional logic to drive home a point or illustrate an eternal truth. He would say things like "the first shall be last," "the humble will be exalted," "the least among you will become the greatest," "the way to live is to die to yourself," "the way to become ruler is to be the servant of all" and so on.

These don't make sense at all to our human reasoning! How can we obtain victory by surrendering? Because that's simply how the Kingdom of heaven operates. We gain a key insight into the nature and function of the eternally wise and all-knowing, all-powerful, everywhere-present creator of the universe from the Old Testament prophet Isaiah. In chapter 55, verse 8 God explains to Isaiah "I don't think the way you think. The way you work isn't the way I work" (MSG). Truly His thought and ways are far above ours.

The Apostle Paul also employs this principle of paradox by helping us understand a key dynamic of the recovery process. In 2 Corinthians 12:7-10, while discussing his painful dilemma regarding an ongoing personal struggle he could not conquer in his own strength, he heard God's still, small voice whisper to him: "'My grace is sufficient for you, for my power is made perfect in weakness.' Therefore I will boast all the more gladly about my weaknesses, so that Christ's power may rest on me...for when I am weak, then I am strong" (NIV).

The power of strength being produced by getting in touch with and acknowledging the reality of our weakness has always been a key feature to recovery. "We didn't stumble into this fellowship brimming with love, honesty, open-mindedness, or willingness....**When we were beaten, we became willing**" (Basic Text, p. 20).

I (Paul) have an inscribed copy of "The Jabez Prayer" sitting on my desk at work, and I read it every day and pray it often during the day. It is listed as a great prayer in I Chronicles 4:10, where a godly man named Jabez prays for God to expand his "territory," which I take to mean his financial possessions as well as his sphere of influence. I pray for God's blessings on me both by blessing me and our non-profit national chain of Meier Clinics, as well as by blessing my ministry opportunities, including blessing this book to help many others. Like Jabez, I pray for God's hand to be upon me, guiding me and blessing me.

But the prayer ends with a very important concept. Jabez prays for God to please help him not to sin—to surrender to God's will rather than to his own sinful nature—so that he will not cause pain to himself and others. When we sin, to be sure there is momentary pleasure or else sin would not be tempting. But in the long run, sin always results in pain to ourselves and others.

Sins all hurt someone. When we cling to our private or "secret sins," we are choosing to inflict pain on ourselves and others, and are being very foolish. Surrender is a necessary part of recovery, but most of us fight it. Much of the pain in our lives comes from fighting and not surrendering. The desire to control people, places, and things causes anxiety, stress, and a feeling of loss of control. Won't you give them up today?

Daily Surrender and Reflection

Please spend a few moments silently reflecting on the spiritual principle of Surrender. Is there a surrender I need to make today? Use the below space to journal about the need for surrender in your life.

_____

_____

_____

_____

_____

_____

_____

_____

_____

_____

_____

_____

_____

_____

DAY TWO

Word of the Day: *Childlike*

Scripture: "He called a little child to him, and placed the child among them. And he said: "Truly I tell you, unless you change and become like little children, you will never enter the kingdom of heaven. Therefore, whoever takes the lowly position of this child is the greatest in the kingdom of heaven. And whoever welcomes one such child in my name welcomes me." (Matthew 18:2-5, NIV)

Quote: "Come to the feet of Jesus knowing you have nothing to offer him." (Pastor Philip Dvorak)

Run to God Like a Little Child

Jesus told the crowd around him, "I tell you the truth, unless you turn from your sins and become like little children, you will never get into the Kingdom of Heaven" (Matthew 18:3, [version?]). What could Jesus possibly mean by this?

I (Phil) am a father of four little ones. Over the years, my wife and I have learned a few things about little children. First, very little children have nothing of worldly value to offer you. They can't get a job, dress themselves, bathe themselves, feed themselves and in fact they are horrible decision makers. My son would decide to eat ice cream three meals a day if we let him (yet he's lactose intolerant). My daughter would eat chocolate incessantly (but she's allergic to chocolate). Children left to care for themselves would not live healthy lives. In fact, most would become unhealthy and die. So what is Jesus saying when he says, "become like little children"?

First, I believe Jesus is saying come to him with nothing to offer. Come to the feet of Jesus knowing you have nothing to offer Him, in humility, broken and empty. He is God and has everything; you come to Him recognizing that you are like a little child who is completely dependent upon Him. For those of us on this journey of addiction recovery, this is a game changing thought. When we realized:

> "...we had to quit playing God. It didn't work. Next, we decided that hereafter in this drama of life, God was going to be our Director. He is the Principal; we are His agents. He is the Father and we are His children. Most good ideas are simple, and this concept was the keystone of the new and triumphant arch through which we passed to freedom." AA p.62

We come to Him in total surrender, total dependence, like a little child.

Second, I believe Jesus is saying come to Him with a childlike faith. Every day when I return from work, as I approach the door, I can hear a stampede ensue on the other side of the door along with, "Daddy's home! Daddy's home! Daddy's home!" Before I'm able to get the door completely open, my children jump on top of me and nearly knock me to the ground with their embrace. My children simply want more of their Daddy. When we finally approach God like a child, we begin to realize the void inside of us we've been trying to fill with drinking or drugging can only truly be satisfied by more of our Heavenly Father. Run to God today like a little child with exuberant and reckless abandon--He is completely safe and trustworthy--unlike many of our earthly parents. He is delighted to scoop us up in His strong and loving arms to comfort and secure us.

Third, little children are completely open, honest and transparent. They don't play mental or emotional games with themselves or others. What you see is what you get. They don't hide, except when playing peek-a-boo or hide and seek; and these are not intended to be self-protective or manipulative. In the same way, God wants us to be real with Him and bring Him our needs, our fears and our vulnerabilities. Again, Jesus is entirely safe, trustworthy and accepting, looking past our faults and seeing our needs.

When we think of "addictions" we traditionally think about alcohol and drugs. But all of us, including myself (Paul) probably have some addictive tendencies of our own, even if we do not drink to excess or abuse drugs. We must all eat, for example, to stay alive, but do we eat to live or live to eat? All of us who are overweight have an addiction problem with food, where we eat food to excess to our own detriment. Your own addictive tendencies may be for attention, lust, or even to be what we call "codependent" where you are addicted to enabling someone else who has an addiction or who takes advantage of your relative inability to say no, even when you should say no.

No matter what our addictive tendencies or all out addictions may be, our basic human nature is to overestimate our ability to look in a mirror (figuratively or literally), see our addiction, and simply decide to quit it that day in our own strength. We may even succeed for a while. But if we rely simply on our own strength, we are doomed to fail. Infants grow up, and little by little, they learn to dress themselves, to feed themselves, to care for themselves, and even to become responsible adults and earn a living and become good parents and citizens in our society. But it is a gradual process, with much guidance along the say.

Like Phil, I (Jared) have four children--all sons. When they were toddlers (which was quite a while ago given that they are all now taller than me), it was cute to see them make initially feeble efforts to become autonomous in varying ways. When one of our guys was about two, we were working outside together one beautiful spring day and he innocently asked what the word "independent" meant. Surprised he was curious about such a big word for a little guy, I tried to explain it in such a way that a small child could grasp the concept, which was hard for me to do. He listened carefully, thought about it for a moment, and exclaimed "Dad, let's be independent together!"

Though amusing to me at that young stage of development, the Bible teaches that all of us eventually rebel and defiantly turn from our childlike innocence to go our own way (Isaiah 53:6). An expression all our boys voiced around the "terrific twos" stage was: "Let me do it my own self."

Children must certainly become independent in healthy ways at the right times and for the right reasons. Yet the charm and warmth of being "independent together" for all of us eventually degenerates into a loss of relationship, caused by the separation resulting from our sinful, shameful, selfish attitudes and actions.

Therefore, we must each come like little children to Jesus, asking Him for the guidance and training and unconditional love and grace and permission to learn from our daily failures. We all sin and thus naturally are afraid of judgment, shame, criticism, and condemnation. He not only does not reject us, He marvelously restores our relationship to Him and delights in us as dearly and deeply loved children.

As adults, we benefit by taking our addictions to Him as well, like little helpless children, seeking His guidance and support. Daily meditation on his love letter to us, the Bible, is something I (Paul) have done almost daily since the age of 10, more than 60 years ago. When I fail, and I still do quite often, passages of scripture come back to me that I may have memorized decades ago to help me with whatever my struggle might be that day.

Daily Surrender and Reflection

Please spend a few moments silently reflecting on your faith. Do you falsely and futility try to earn God's love, by attempting to prove you have something to offer him? Like a little child do you simply long for more of your heavenly Father? How can you practice running to God like a little child? Is there anything you need to surrender in order to increase your faith? Use the below space to respond to these questions and journal your thoughts.

_____

_____

_____

_____

_____

_____

_____

_____

_____

_____

_____

_____

_____

DAY THREE

Word of the Day: *Community*

Scripture: "A person standing alone can be attacked and defeated, but two can stand back-to-back and conquer. Three are even better, for a triple-braided cord is not easily broken." (Ecclesiastes 4:12, NLT)

Quote: "Of the thousands of individuals I have worked with struggling with addiction, I have never seen one of them recover alone." (Pastor Philip Dvorak)

It's Not Good For Man To Be Alone

The story of creation starts off with a list of things that are good. Then God said, "Let there be light" (Genesis 1:3), and there was light. God saw that the light was good. God called the dry land earth, and the gathering of the waters He called seas; and God saw that it was good.

However, the list of good things ends, followed by the first thing that God says isn't good. God stated, "It's not good for man to be alone" (Genesis 2:18). You see, deep inside every person, God has placed an inherent need for connection with others—a need for deep, meaningful and fulfilling relationships.

We live in a society that on the surface is seemingly connected. I can read on Facebook about how my college roommate got new carpet in his house (it was really ugly; he always had strange taste), or how it was 100 degrees at my grandmother's house in Arizona today (and how that is unusually tepid for this time of year). However, I haven't sat with either of these people in over a decade. I have a false sense of closeness that at times seems to lead to greater isolation. I no longer know my neighbors and they no longer know me. How can we love our neighbors if we don't know them? God exists in community (Father, Son and Holy Spirit); it is essential that we create and dwell in true community.

Addiction can have some of the most potentially devastating effects on community. Our behavior as an addict/alcoholic hurts not only us, but everyone who is connected to us. As a result, it becomes nearly impossible for others to maintain a close connection to us. Addiction tills some of the most fertile ground for isolation.

You might remember learning about B.F. Skinner and the Skinner Box studies back in middle school and high school. We learned much of our current conception of addiction from these studies. Place a single rat in a box and give it the choice between water and water laced with an addictive substance, and over time the rat would drink the laced water until they died. These studies rightly showed the amazing power of addiction.

However, another study often referred to as Rat Park showed an additional perspective. Alexander and Fraser felt that maybe the box itself played a role in the results, so they created Rat Park. They placed the rats in a more "enjoyable" environment and more importantly, placed other rats with them. The results were truly amazing. For the most part, the rats then chose the plain water over the water laced with the addictive substance. When the rats were isolated they drank the laced water to the grave, but when in community they were much more likely to thrive.

Satan and your addiction like to isolate you. The more isolated you become, the easier it is to destroy you. It is as if you are living in one of Skinner's cages. You will begin to drink the laced water. In the thousands of individuals I (Phil) have worked with struggling with addiction, I have never seen one of them recover alone. They found connection again through counseling, 12-step fellowships, and church community.

One thing I (Paul) have found to be particularly helpful in creating community in my own life is to have a prayer partner. I have had numerous prayer partners throughout my adult life, and have several now. But I always have one primary prayer partner who I go to in order to confess a sin I recently committed, or to ask for advice, or to request prayer, or just to share my life with. We even send jokes to each other sometimes by email.

My prayer partner for over thirty years was a fellow Christian Psychiatrist, Dr. Dave Larson, a researcher in the area of the effects of religious beliefs and practices on mental and physical health. He was an exceptionally godly man, and it was usually me confessing to him.

In 2002, my great friend Dave died suddenly from an aortic aneurysm and beat me to Heaven. I missed him deeply and still do. I prayed for God to guide me in finding another primary prayer partner to replace Dave. I knew it had to be a male, because I do not think anyone should have that close of a relationship to anyone of the opposite sex other than his or her mate, because Satan can use even a good relationship to turn sour into an emotional or physical affair.

A decade earlier, I had been on a missionary trip to Israel. My son went with me, but had to fly home earlier than me for his college, so I flew home alone. On the first leg of my flight, from Tel Aviv to Paris, nobody spoke English on either side of me so I had nobody to talk to, which is hard on an ADHD person like myself. The next flight was going to be over seven hours long, from Paris to Chicago, so I prayed that God would put someone beside me who spoke at least broken English and was willing to talk with me.

A young woman from Paris sat beside me and spoke decent English, so I thanked God and struck up a conversation. We only shared our first names at first, and I found out that she (Katherine) was going to Little Rock, Arkansas to visit a woman who had been a missionary to Paris ten years earlier, when Katherine was a college student in Paris and was going through a deep depression from breaking up with her fiancé. The missionary from Little Rock gave Katherine a book at the time, and Katherine asked me if I had ever heard of the book. It was <u>Happiness is a Choice</u>, by Dr. Paul Meier.

I did not tell her that I am Paul Meier, but said I had heard about that book. She said as a result of reading that book, she not only got over her depression but became a Christian and now was a missionary herself to college students in the Paris area. Katherine went on to tell me she was going to Little Rock to visit the missionary who gave her that book, but also to hunt down Dr. Paul Meier to get his advice on how the other missionaries there in Paris could get training in Christian psychology.

To her shock, I pulled out my passport and showed her that I am Paul Meier and asked her when she would like me to fly to Paris to train her group. A few months later, I was in Paris, training her group, along with a Christian Psychologist from Paris by the name of Dr. Jean-Luc Bertrand. He and I became good friends and even visited each other over the years to come. So when Dave Larson died in 2002, after much prayer, I decided to ask Jean Luc if he would be my prayer partner, doing so by email most of the time. He asked me why I would want someone in Paris to be my prayer partner all the way in Dallas, Texas.

I told him there were three reasons: 1. He lived thousands of miles away so it was easier to confess personal sins to him and not worry about gossip getting out; 2. He was a Christian Psychologist and I was a Christian Psychiatrist, so we could analyze each other to see why we are tempted more in certain areas of our lives than other areas; and 3. My earlier prayer partner, Dave, was so godly if was almost always me confessing to him, and I knew that since Jean Luc was French, he must sin at least as much as I do!! He laughed and said he was definitely qualified in that regard and we became prayer partners ever since. When I am tempted daily to sin, it is much easier for me to resist knowing I will only have to admit it to my friend short time later. There is strength in community.

I (Phil) see miracles on a daily basis. People who were taking their last sips of that tainted water reach out for help, and I get to watch as God restores their lives. It is not good for any of us to be alone. Don't spend another day growing more and more isolated; reach out today. I promise you that you will not have to do this alone. Call a sober support, share with a prayer partner, go to a meeting, attend church, or perform some service work.

Why encourage church involvement as part of recovery? Outside of the scriptural reasons to encourage involvement in a church (e.g., Hebrews 10:25), let's look at the research. According to the research of Kendler, M.D., and Myers, M.S. from the American Psychiatric Association, church attendance is one of the most consistent predictors of abstinence from substance use.

The 2009 study compared nearly 2,000 sets of twins for over six years and found that there was an inverse relationship between church attendance and substance abuse. They also found that the inverse relationship grew stronger over time. In other words, as a person's church attendance became more consistent the less likely they were to abuse substances. Becoming a part of a church home can be one of the best ways you can be supported in your continued sobriety. And as important as recovery supports and groups are, don't let the rooms of recovery become your church.

"A Sheep Alone Dies." I was told this once by a pastor friend and I never forgot it. He stated that you can put a sheep in the best pasture, but without companionship it will almost certainly die. A sheep needs community to thrive.

Throughout the Scriptures God's children are often referred to as sheep; sheep who have gone astray, sheep being placed at the right hand of Jesus. We, like sheep, need community. If we are going to live a full, abundant, sober life, we need the support and encouragement of others. Seek a deep friendship and eternal relationship with the true Creator God and "hang out" with fellow believers who are like minded in their view of God and his Word.

Please be reminded today that you can't fight this battle alone. Each of us needs a community of people to lean on. Find a meeting, find a sponsor, and get involved in a church. Don't try to fight this disease without the support of others.

Daily Surrender and Reflection

Please spend a few moments silently reflecting on your need for community. In what ways has your addiction impacted your connection to others? Do you avoid community? If so why? What are some ways you can better develop community in your life? Do you have a healthy church? Are you known there--are you involved in a small group and ministry there? Who is your sponsor, pastor, prayer partner, mentor or sober friends? Use the below space to answer these questions and journal about your thoughts.

_____

_____

_____

_____

_____

_____

_____

_____

_____

_____

_____

_____

_____

DAY FOUR

Words of the Day: *Knowing God*

Scripture: "And this is eternal life, that they know you the only true God, and Jesus Christ whom you have sent." (John 17:3 ESV)

Quote: "He is the great I Am. Jesus is not simply a higher power, He is the highest power."(Pastor Philip Dvorak)

Be Still and Know that I Am God

"Be still and know that I am God" (Psalm 46:10, NIV). This verse has been popularized in our culture today. Popularized might be too kind; I (Phil) think "hijacked" might be more appropriate. The verse in today's culture means to slow down, to stop striving. So far, so good. But the "know that I am God" part has been interpreted to mean such things as "All is God and God is in all", "Find the God within", and "Become one with the universal energy". These statements are far from what this scripture was intended to mean.

Psalm 46:1-3 says, "God is our refuge and strength, an ever-present help in trouble. Therefore we will not fear, though the earth gives way and the mountains fall into the heart of the sea, though its waters roar and foam and the mountains quake with their surging" (NIV). Later in the chapter, the psalmist says, 'Be still, and know that I am God; I will be exalted among the nations, I will be exalted in the earth.' The Lord Almighty is with us; the God of Jacob is our fortress" (10-11).

Our culture, for the most part, has the first part of this verse correct. Surrender to the fact that God is in control and stop striving. Be still. However, God is not some force we can manipulate to fulfill our selfish desires and needs. He is the great I Am. He is not simply a higher power, He is the highest power. The "know" part of this verse is ultimate intimacy. To "know" God is a translation of the Hebrew word Yada, which means to fully know and to be fully known. It's to fully recognize who God is and who we are in relationship to God. When we know God in this way, it changes everything.

"The Four C's" of knowing God:

when we know God, He:

1) **Calms Us** - Satan wants to confuse us. The great deceiver wants to distract us from truly knowing God, but God wants to give the weary rest (Matthew 11:28). When we know God and know that he will never leave us or forsake us, no matter what storms we are facing, the knowledge that God is with us will give us a peace that surpasses all understanding (Philippians 4:7).

2) **Convicts Us** - Knowing God gives us the great gift of conviction. When we know who God is, we are convicted by our sin. He convicts us NOT to shame us, but to teach us in a better way to live and think. He guides us in a way that brings more love and joy and peace and meaning in our lives. When we truly reflect on the perfect character of God, we can't help but see our sins and have godly sorrow. Satan, however, tries to conceal our sin, and tries to convince us that our sins aren't really sins. If he fails at that, he tries to convince us that our sins are unforgivable and that we are permanently defeated and worthless. The sickness concealed just gets infected and makes us sicker. As the saying goes in Alcoholics Anonymous, "you are only as sick as your secrets."

3) **Compels Us to Change** - Knowing God convicts us, which then compels us to change. 2 Corinthians 5:14 says, "For Christ's love compels us…" (NIV). Knowing who God is and that He loved us to the point of dying on the cross should compel us to live a life

set apart for him. However, Satan will try to speak condemnation into our lives, in an attempt to cage us to our past. Knowing God will remind us "there is no condemnation for those in Christ Jesus," says Romans 8:1 (NIV). Truly knowing God will compel us to change.

4) **Courage to Continue** - Knowing God gives us courage to continue. "Though the earth give way and the mountains fall into the heart of the sea..." (NIV] Knowing that the great I Am will never leave us nor forsake us should give us courage--courage to face the inevitable storms of this life. God has our backs. Psalm 46:6-8 says, "The Lord Almighty is with us; the God of Jacob is our fortress" (NIV). The creator of the universe wants us to know him and He wants to know us. Satan wants us to cower in fear. When we truly know God, we will learn to fear no evil because God is with us.

I (Paul) had a book published in 2015 that I had been working on, little by little, for over eight years, called Knowing God Outside the Box (Morgan James, Publisher, New York). It has a couple hundred pages of advice on how to know the real God intimately, and I urge all the readers of this book to please read that for more depth in this topic. There are seven billion people on planet earth, and we all have at least a slightly different view of who God is, so that proves that we are all at least a little bit wrong, since God is God and we can't invent him in our minds and hearts.

We learn from psychiatry research that much of our God concept is tainted by whatever our earthly fathers are like, for example. When, as a three year old, we learn to pray to our Heavenly Father, what we are really thinking is "Dear Heavenly Version of my earthly father..." If we have a harsh and condemning father, we tend to see God that way. If we have a father who spoils us we tend to become "name it, claim it" Christians who get up in the morning with our prayers consisting of a "to do" list for God to do everything for us and to indulge us with our selfish desires. If we have an absent father, we tend to think there is no God, or that if there is one, he is off at a distance not really caring about us personally.

There are a host of other obstacles that can keep us from knowing God intimately, the way He really is, rather than the way we falsely imagine

Him to be. There are religions that teach you exactly how you should see God to be like, and if you differ from their dogma, you can, in some cases, even be killed. Take ISIS in Iraq and Syria for example. We must think for ourselves and not let someone else dictate to us what the true God is like.

The true God is the God of the Bible, and Jesus is His one and only "...Son [who] is the radiance of God's glory and the exact representation of his being..." (Hebrews 1:3, NIV). If we really want to know who and what and how God really is, study His Word. Jesus Himself explained to us that "If you really know me, you will know my Father as well" (John 14:7). So studying the Bible is a great way to get to know the real God better, but sometimes people even misquote the Bible or say it is saying something it really isn't saying. So pray for the real God to make himself known to you and search for the real Creator God.

Daily Surrender and Reflection

tPlease spend a few moments to be still and know that He is God and reflect on how knowing God changes everything? How is he calming you, convicting you, compelling you to change, and giving you the courage to change? Use the below space to journal about what it means to know God.

_____

_____

_____

_____

_____

_____

_____

_____

_____

_____

_____

_____

_____

DAY FIVE

Word of the Day: *Loving*

Scripture: "Love the Lord your God with all your heart and with all your soul and with all your mind. This is the first and greatest commandment. And the second is like it: Love your neighbor as yourself. All the Law and the Prophets hang on these two commandments." (Matthew 22:37-40, NIV)

Quote: "The rules that are intended to help us live safely and freely have ironically begun to imprison us." (Pastor Philip Dvorak)

Don't Do That

I (Phil) live in a beautiful home in an immaculate neighborhood. We've truly been blessed to have the home we do; however, our neighborhood has a fairly restrictive homeowners association (HOA). Everywhere you turn you see signs posted touting rule after rule, telling us what we can't do as well as what we must do. Yet, it seems with each passing year another problem arises and the HOA simply adds a new sign with a few more don'ts. Everywhere I turn it seems like another restriction has been placed on what we are able to do. No fishing, no swimming, no running, no skateboarding, no parking and the list goes on and on. Most of these rules have good intentions (though some I think are ludicrous), but most of them are there to keep our community safe, secure, and attractive.

However, these rules have become almost overwhelming. In fact, there are so many don'ts now that at times I'm confused about what exactly we can do, to the point that it now seems nearly impossible to keep all the rules. My neighbor is a sheriff and his cruiser was towed out of his driveway in the middle of the night (because "commercial" vehicles are not allowed). My wife rode with a friend to a dinner party and when she returned, she realized she didn't have her driver's license. She was not allowed to enter the neighborhood until I was able to find a neighbor to watch our kids, so that I could take her picture ID to the guard gate. We have friends who cringe when we invite them to come over because they dread waiting in line to get through the security gate.

Another amenity we enjoy in our neighborhood is a gorgeous resort-style community pool. The "don'ts" say that we can only have up to four guests per family. One of our closest family friends is fostering two children and has two children of their own. Because they are fostering these children, they are no longer allowed to enjoy the blessing of our pool as a family. The rules that are intended to help us live safely and freely have ironically begun to imprison us.

Similar to the HOA in my neighborhood, recovery and religion can easily become restrictive or even oppressive cultures of don'ts. Don't smoke, don't dance, don't dress like that, don't have sex outside of marriage, don't lie, don't steal, don't pierce that, don't drink that, don't eat that, don't listen to that, don't watch that and the list goes on and on. Don't misunderstand me here. Although some of these don'ts are legalistic, most of these don'ts are vitally important and our families, communities, and our society would be safer if we kept them. However, I can get lost in the don'ts at times and miss the most important do's.

Two thousand years ago, Jesus lived in a religious culture of don'ts. The Ten Commandments had become hundreds upon hundreds of commandments. It became literally impossible to keep track of all the don'ts. He was approached by the religious experts of the time and asked an impossible question in Matthew 22:36, "Teacher, which is the great commandment in the Law" (NIV)? Of all these rules which one do we really need to make sure we keep? Jesus response is brilliantly succinct. Jesus replied, "Love the Lord your God with all your heart and with all your soul and with all your mind. This is the first and greatest commandment. And the second is like it: Love your neighbor as yourself. All the Law and the Prophets hang on these two commandments." (Matthew 22:37-40, NIV).

Jesus turns the list of hundreds and hundreds of don'ts into three simple do's. Love God, love your neighbors, and love yourself; do this and all the other laws will fall into place. We all miss the mark; we all will mess up and break some of the don'ts. My challenge today is for each of us to stop being overwhelmed by the don'ts and keep it simple and focus on these three do's. How well are you doing at loving God? Loving your neighbor? Loving yourself? I'm going to spend a little more time focusing on these three do's and trust Jesus. He says if I keep these three, the rest of the don'ts will fall into place.

We understand that loving God means to really develop a deep relationship with the One True Creator God, the God of the Bible, not some father-projection or imaginary God your earlier religion may have shoved down your throat. And to obey the Great Commandment, we must also love our neighbors as we love ourselves.

Some legalistic religions teach that it is a sin to love yourself. This can be confusing or controversial to some because it is sinful to be a selfish narcissist, putting your own desires higher than others to the detriment of others. But the truth is we cannot love anyone else more or better than we love ourselves. We simply can't give what we don't have. It is a natural law of physics that a stream cannot rise higher than its source. So to it is a natural human law of relationship that we are to love our neighbor as we love ourselves.

But we must learn to love ourselves as God graciously loves us. We have to allow the Lord to fill our own love tanks before we will have enough love in them to spill out and share that love with others.

To love someone else is to love and care for what is best for that other person, to the point of self-sacrifice if necessary. If you "fall in love" romantically with someone else who doesn't not love you back, then you will not get angry at the other person who does not feel romantically toward you. If you truly love that other person, you will want whatever is best for that other person, even if it is not you. Loving our neighbors is wanting what is best for them. Introducing them to a relationship with God is always a loving thing to do, but must be done in a loving way.

Daily Surrender and Reflection

Please spend a few moments answering these three questions; How well are you doing at loving God, loving your neighbor, and loving yourself? Use the below space to answer these questions and to journal about how you could improve your love for God, neighbor and yourself.

DAY SIX

Word of the Day: *Anger*

Scripture: "People with understanding control their anger; a hot temper shows great foolishness." (Proverbs 14:29, NLT)

Quote: "God wants us to be like him. He is slow to anger."(Pastor Philip Dvorak)

In Your Anger Do Not Sin

We live in an angry world. Did you get angry today? As we look around us, we can't avoid the anger in this world. Turn on the news. Drive on the highway, and you will witness if not experience someone's "road rage." From wars around the world, to wars in our homes, we are living in some really angry times.

Ephesians 4:26 challenges us to "Be angry, and do not sin" (NIV). Be angry. That statement presumes that we will get what? Angry. Everyone gets angry. It's human nature. God gets angry and we are made in his image--He just doesn't sin in His anger. Some of our anger is righteous indignation toward someone who is lying about us or sinning against us.

Some of our anger is inappropriate, because of our pride or paranoia. In the original Greek, Ephesians 4:26 is written in the passive-imperative sense, meaning to "go ahead and get angry (at appropriate times implied) without sinning." It is a quote from Psalm 4:4 which directs us to "Be angry, and do not sin" (ESV). However, what we do with our anger is what really matters.

In our anger we should not sin. If we're slapping our kids and spouse around in anger, we've got a problem. If we react to our feelings in such a manner that we're cussing at people whenever we have a disagreement, we have a problem. If we are getting angry because we are being selfish or perfectionistic or overly suspicious, we have a problem.

What we do with our anger and other feelings directly affects our sobriety and our interpersonal relationships. Anger can motivate you to change. Stuffed anger is one of the leading causes of depression and addictions. You are more tempted to lust when you are angry at your mate, for example.

You can get angry at the injustice in the world, and do something about it. If you see someone beating a child, your anger can motivate you to stop them. By the same token, you can get angry at the disease of addiction. This righteous anger can motivate a positive change in you. This change can impact your life and the lives of all those with who, you come into contact.

But for me (Jared), consistently living out the life-giving principles regarding anger embedded within James 1:19 is very challenging. Jesus' half-brother teaches us we should "Understand this, my beloved brothers and sisters. Let everyone be quick to hear [be a careful, thoughtful listener], slow to speak [a speaker of carefully chosen words and], slow to anger [patient, reflective, forgiving]" (AMP). In my own flesh and strength, I tend to be tempted to do the exact opposite of these three fundamental principles of spiritual, psychological and relational health. It's easy for me to reactively be slow to hear, quick to speak and quick to become angry.

Like many people, much of my anger is reactive in nature. When I react, the fruit of the Holy Spirit is not evidenced or applied, especially the fruit of self-control (Galatians 5: 22-23). But when I refuse to be defensive or self-protective and allow the Holy Spirit to guide and direct me, I can listen to the still small voice of God (1 Kings 19:12) and *respond* according to James 1:19 rather than *react* sinfully according to my human nature.

Psychologically we know that most human anger is an unconscious reaction to attempt to empower oneself (albeit falsely) when we experience a deeper emotion which is too threatening to experience or express in a healthy way. Consequently, generally we become angry instead of facing the underlying sense of fear, helplessness, powerlessness, hurt or vulnerability.

We often subconsciously try to trick ourselves into feeling powerful and enraged (which instantly releases a host of intense biochemical changes into our bloodstream and neurological pathways) instead of feeling the denied sense of powerlessness, fear and/or hurt.

Over the last several years, one of the things I have been most impressed by in my personal study of Jesus' identity, personality and interpersonal relationship dynamics is that *He never once reacted to anyone or anything.* That is absolutely stunning! I see so many ways in which I unconsciously allow other people to push my buttons or frustrate me in some way, often tempting me to be reactive instead of responsive. And in every case, my immaturity in those situations gives my personal power away to the other person.

Jesus always responded. He never reacted. Jesus was always fully and maturely in complete self-control. He was able to say with authority "This is why the Father loves me: because I freely lay down my life. And so I am free to take it up again. No one takes it from me. I lay it down of my own free will…" (John 10:17, MSG). When we exercise our free will and do not react to whatever others do or don't do, we don't have any childish temper fits. We don't cut people off in traffic, and we don't yell at those who cut us off. Consequently, we also don't have to take as much blood pressure, migraine headache or stomach ulcer medicine!

Let's look at what Psalm 103:8 says to us about these truths: "The LORD is merciful and gracious, slow to anger, and abounding in mercy" (NKJV). God wants us to be like Him. He is slow to anger. He wants us to be slow to anger. He doesn't need to prove Himself. He is secure in who He is and the Almighty simply chooses to, amidst the chaos of this world, speak calmly and quietly, in a still small voice.

But you know who tries to roar? The devil shows us his teeth and roars in an attempt to intimidate. You see the devil in his pride, in his insecurities, tries to prove to himself, and convince us, that he is more powerful than our God. But, it simply isn't true.

God, who is infinitely more powerful, doesn't need to prove anything to anyone. He simply whispers. Let's all try to remember this the next time we get angry. We don't have to show our teeth to anyone. We can simply let go and let God.

When we react impulsively in our anger, we are reacting with the anger of man. But when we slow down, and seek God in the midst of our anger, we listen to God's still small voice. Then, we can respond in a righteous way, rather than an impulsive, sinful way. Remember Proverbs 14:29: people with understanding control their anger; a hot temper shows great foolishness. Let's not be foolish. Let us be slow to anger, and abound in mercy today.

Daily Surrender and Reflection

Please spend a few moments reflecting on your anger. How has your anger put your recovery at risk? Are you slow to anger? Do you sin in your anger? How can you more fully surrender reacting to your anger and learn to respond? How are you at abounding in mercy? What is your righteous anger motivating you to change? Use the below space to answer these questions and to journal about how you could improve how you respond to your anger.

_____

_____

_____

_____

_____

_____

_____

_____

_____

_____

_____

_____

_____

_____

DAY SEVEN

Word of the Day: *Faith*

Scripture: "Faith is the confidence that what we hope for will actually happen; it gives us assurance about things we cannot see." (Hebrews 11:1, NLT)

Quote: "Do you want to believe? Maybe that's enough to start." (Pastor Philip Dvorak)

Overcoming Unbelief

Many of us have this false belief that we have to have it all figured out before we can approach God. We feel guilty for doubting. However, God can handle our questions and our doubts.

One of my (Phil) favorite scriptures is Mark 9:24 which says "...I do believe, help my unbelief!" (NIV).. Here is a man who is standing face to face with Jesus Christ and he still suffers with doubts—with unbelief. Do you have any doubts? Maybe you need to cut yourself some slack. This father had a child who was tormented spiritually and physically. His son was suffering from horrific seizures that would render him deaf and mute. During these seizures the child would often fall into fire and water. He would be burning alive and couldn't cry out for help or hear those trying to help him. The father wanted his son to be well. He loved his son. This was his only child. The child was the man's blessing, his legacy. And he came to Christ imploring "Teacher, I beg you, look at my son, my only child." I beg you. Please help me.

This father is desperate. Like any good father, he wants more than anything for his son to be well, for the torment to end and he hears of Jesus. He thinks, I'm willing to do anything to see my son get well. Maybe this Jesus and his followers can help. He finds Jesus' disciples and begs them to heal his boy. And they fail! The men closest to Jesus were not able to heal his son.

I can only imagine the doubt that was creeping in this father's mind. Why can't they heal my son? What do I have to do? I want to believe, but I doubt. I want more than anything to believe you can heal my child.

How much faith do you have? Do you want to believe? Maybe that's enough to start. So in absolute desperation this father begs Jesus to look at his son. Look at him as he foams at the mouth—look at his scars, his burns, please, I beg you. Please, Jesus, can you can heal my boy? Of course this father doubted. Who wouldn't? The pain has been more real than any healing. All he has known for years is this bondage, is the suffering of his son. He was so much more acquainted with the struggle than with the victory. He wants it to be true, but the doctors have failed, the rabbis, the faith healers, all have failed. Nothing has worked.

For many of us who are hurt by the disease of addiction, all we can remember is the suffering. You've tried so many different things and nothing seems to work. For years your family has been in bondage to the addiction. What do you do? Do you give up in despair and unbelief? Do you let your doubts take over and stop you from pursuing after God? Or do you respond like this father? I love this father's response. It's so sincere. It's so brutally honest. It's so real. I believe, Jesus, help me overcome my unbelief. "I do believe, but help me overcome my unbelief!"

This father wants more than anything in the world to believe. To believe that Jesus is who he says he is. Because if he is, than he can certainly heal this son. If he is truly the long awaited promised Messiah, if he is the Son of the living God, if he is the great "I Am," then nothing is impossible for him. If Jesus is who he claims to be, he can restore us to our sanity. With his help we can overcome the bondages of addiction.

This man in the Biblical story is, like any of us in desperate circumstances, understandably gripped by fear. I (Jared) can deeply identify with and relate to this father's fearful sense of paternal love and complete helplessness. I will never forget the day when the chief of

Pediatric Oncology at Children's Mercy Hospital in Kansas City looked across his desk and said to my wife Linda and me; "Your son has Acute Lymphoblastic Leukemia." Like this man, we wanted to have faith, but in our fear we also knew at that time this particular diagnosis was almost a certain death sentence.

Over the next forty months of his chemo treatment, we watched all but our then three year old son and one other boy from their original 29 member treatment protocol group tragically pass away (then the other boy unexpectedly relapsed five years after treatment and died within two weeks). During that grueling, grievous and grotesque season of fear, our faith was stretched and challenged in many painful and traumatic ways.

Among the many powerful lessons I learned from those torturous long three and a third years is that *faith is the opposite of fear.* Our son nearly died three times the first year. There were situations, complications and circumstances where we were very afraid, yet we exercised our faith. The truth is unless we courageously face our fears head on, our faith does not grow. It is easy for our human fear to grab us by the throat and get in the way of our faith development. But in the Biblical account, this man's desperation led him instead to believe. And so did we.

I also learned much about suffering as we watched all those precious little bald-headed kids lose their valiant struggle against the scourge of cancer. I used to think the book of Job was about suffering. But I no longer do--I believe the predominant theme and message of Job is about faith.

Listen to this great patriarch's expression of his deep and unwavering faith in the midst of the most dire, dreadful and drastic circumstances imaginable: "Though He slay me, yet will I trust Him" (Job 13:15, NKJV). The profound truth I realized about fearful and painful things in life from his story is this: *faith like Job's cannot be shaken, because faith like Job's is the result of having been shaken.* Faith cancels out fear.

Perhaps you've heard the old sermon illustration that the word "fear" can be understood by the acronym: False Evidence Appearing Real. The scriptures repeatedly tell us to not be afraid because it is entirely normal and natural--but not healthy or holy--to be consumed by fear when our faith is weak or wavering. God wants to transform our fears into faith. Miraculously in the process, we grow, and He is glorified.

Many years ago, a Christian recording artist named Andre Crouch wrote a powerful and popular song called "Through it All." It boldly and bravely addressed our fears, problems and difficulties in an honest but redemptive way. He pointed out that if we never had problems, we would never know God could solve them. The refrain assures us that through it all, we can learn to trust in Jesus and learn to depend upon His Word.

I (Paul) have patients come from all over the world to our Day Programs, and I evaluate the ones who come to our Dallas clinic. They stay at a hotel nearby and come to our clinic for about seven hours a day, five days a week, for about three weeks. We pack six months to a year of therapy into those three weeks, digging and probing for root problems and resolving them to bring about healing from a host of psychiatric problems, most often depression.

I remember when a new patient named David came to our Day Program and I began his treatment with a one hour evaluation. David was suicidally depressed, had panic attacks, and had several different addiction problems. He was a committed Christian, but never had therapy.

The Bible says that in a multitude of counselors there is safety, but David always tried to quit his addictions on his own. He would repent, do well for a while, and then fail again. He had finally lost faith in himself, and to be honest, he needed to. We can't make it on our own. He wondered if God could still accept him or help him. I showed David Proverbs 24:16, where the Bible tells us that God considers someone who fails seven times in a row but keeps trying a "righteous man." David lacked faith that God still loved him, and lacked faith that God could heal him, but he had a glimmer of faith and hope, and that was the start of his healing. But David had to quit trying on his own and call on the true Higher Power, Jesus Christ, to help him see his root problems and rely on God, on Christian professional counselors, and on getting in touch with his buried and unresolved emotions.

In the weeks to come, David gained many insights into his areas of dependency and buried emotions, and overcame his depression, panic attacks, and his addictions. He realized there would be lifelong temptations to return to his addictive tendencies, and that he would need lifelong support to succeed—groups, a good church, a prayer partner, and sometimes maybe even ongoing therapy. But David did well and grew stronger and stronger spiritually and emotionally. I heard from David many years later, and he and his family were continuing to prosper.

Daily Surrender and Reflection

Please spend a few moments reflecting on your faith and your doubts. Do you have faith? Do you doubt? Do you want to believe? How has your addiction and your recovery impacted your faith? What areas do you need God's help in increasing your faith? Use the below space to answer these questions and to journal about your faith and your doubts.

_____

_____

_____

_____

_____

_____

_____

_____

_____

_____

_____

_____

_____

_____

DAY EIGHT

Word of the Day: *Pride*

Scripture: "When pride comes, then comes disgrace, but with humility comes wisdom." (Proverbs 11:2, NIV)

Quote: "Humility is not thinking less of yourself, it's thinking of yourself less." (C.S. Lewis)

The Blessing of Humility and the Curse of Pride

The 12-steps, and the Big Book of Alcoholics Anonymous are based from the Good Book, the Bible, and in particular the book of James. In fact, the earliest participants in what would later be called AA were often referred to as the "James Club," and they referred to the book of James as essential to their recovery. James 5:16 says that we need to confess our faults to one another in order to be healed. That can happen in group therapy, in a Sunday School class, with a prayer partner, in individual therapy, between husband and wife, and many other ways. But we need to confess our sins and faults not only to God, but to one another in order to experience healing in our lives. One of the best ways for those of us recovering from addiction is working through the steps with a 12-step sponsor.

I (Paul) have had prayer partners throughout my adult life, and will until the day I die. I am far from perfect. I sin just like anyone else does, but when I do, I share my sin with my prayer partner, and he shares his sins with me. We pray for each other. Just knowing when I am tempted to sin that if I yield, I will have to admit it to my prayer partner, keeps me most of the time from committing whatever sin I am tempted to commit that day. I have to humble myself enough to admit my sins and flaws to my good friend and prayer partner.

James the brother of Jesus was very close to Jesus, he was his family and a disciple. He certainly has the right to speak from a position of authority. However, here is what he has to say. "James, a servant of God and of the Lord Jesus Christ" (James 1:1, ESV). James, "a servant". Instead of saying "Hey, I'm the brother of Jesus, you need to listen to what I have to say" James introduces himself as a servant of God and the Lord Jesus Christ. He takes a position of humility. He is humble. Unpretentious. Not full of or stuck on himself.

Just a few chapters later in this same letter, James quotes the Old Testament proverb: "God opposes the proud but shows favor to the humble" (4:6, NIV). When we are in the midst of our addiction we can be some proud crazy people can't we? The scriptures say here that God opposes the proud. If you are in opposition to someone, you're in a battle against them. You're enemies of them. When we are proud, when we are arrogant, we think we know better than the almighty and we are in opposition to God. We are his enemies. I don't know anyone who wants to be an enemy of the almighty God.

Yet the truth is that pride is our universal human default mode of being. None of our (Jared's) four sons had to be taught the words "mine" or "no!" They were each selfish sinners from infancy (though they were all a lot cuter when they were much shorter and looked less like their dad!). And the worst part of is that their propensity to their sinful nature was and is completely genetic.

The essence of our built-in sin nature--from the factory--is to be as God. The Bible helps us understand that we are all selfish sinners (Romans 3:23) and like sheep, we all want to go our own way instead of obey the voice of our Great Shepherd (Isaiah 53:6). That has been true of humans since Genesis chapter 3 where the first couple rebelled against God's only command to proudly want what they wanted when they wanted it because they wanted it. And the curse of sin has followed us all since.

But God shows favor to the humble. When we are humble, he's on our team, he's fighting for us, not against us. He defends us, and does not judge or condemn us (John 3:17; Romans 8:1-2).. He gives us what we do not deserve. He blesses us and lavishes on us grace, love and mercy.

What a profound lesson for recovery! Recovery is not about keeping up appearances. Pride is one of the most dangerous traits for those of us in recovery. We might have a bitter taste in our mouths when we think about being humble, but the rewards of humbling ourselves by asking for help sweetens our recovery. Pride is insisting that our way will work; humility is realizing that our way has not and will not work.

The importance of humility for the recovering alcoholic and addict is without parallel. Unless individuals admit they cannot drink or use and enlist the help of God to conquer their disease, there is little hope that they will survive the brutality and dangerous consequences of their addiction. Pride always seems to go before our fall. In fact, Paul warns us: "...don't be so naive and self-confident. You're not exempt. You could fall flat on your face as easily as anyone else. Forget about self-confidence; it's useless. Cultivate God-confidence" (1 Corinthians 10:12, MSG).

We must destroy our pride. Pride will kill us. Solomon warned us that "Pride goes before destruction, and a haughty spirit before a fall" (Proverbs 16:18, ESV). Pride will make us an adversary of God. We need to humble ourselves.

Jesus himself humbled himself to the point of being spit at, beaten, stripped naked, and nailed to a cross. Philippians chapter two tells us that even though Jesus is God, he was humble enough to become a human, and to suffer death on the cross for our sins. We are instructed in that passage to "let this mind be in you as was also in Christ Jesus" (verse 5, NKJV). We are to humble ourselves even as Jesus did. As people in recovery we must lose the egos, lose the agendas, and get on our faces before God and cry out to him.

The Message version paraphrases Isaiah 2:11 this way: "People with a big head are headed for a fall, pretentious egos brought down a peg." Remember, "Humble yourselves before the Lord, and he will lift you up" (James 4:10 NIV). That's the true and liberating paradox of the recovery process.

Daily Surrender and Reflection

Please spend a few moments silently reflecting on the spiritual principle of humility. In what ways has your addiction impacted the practice of humility in your life? How has your pride caused you to be in opposition to God? Do you still have pride that needs to be humbled? Use the below space to journal about it.

_____

_____

_____

_____

_____

_____

_____

_____

_____

_____

_____

_____

_____

DAY NINE

Word of the Day: Hope

Scripture: "For I know the plans I have for you, declares the Lord, plans to prosper you and not to harm you, plans to give you hope and a future." (Jeremiah 29:11, NIV)

Quote: "God has better plans for us. His eyes see what can be done. He wants to rebuild us." (Pastor Michael Eleveld)

Living in Despair

We get comfortable in our own filth. After the birth of one of our children, life had gotten a little overwhelming. We (Phil's family) just couldn't find time to do that much needed deep cleaning. My father blessed us with a gift of a cleaning service and they spent the entire day cleaning our home from top to bottom. When they were done cleaning I was amazed by how clean things were. More accurately I was amazed at how I had stopped seeing how dirty things had gotten. I knew things were bad, but I had no clue how truly disgusting they had gotten. Sometimes when we are in the middle of filth, the middle of pain, or the middle of despair, we get comfortable and forget how beautiful things can really be.

There is a great story in the Bible about a man named Nehemiah. He was the cupbearer of the king. The Jewish people had been back living in Jerusalem for approximately 100 years. Nehemiah heard about the conditions in Jerusalem, that the walls were still down and the temple had still not been rebuilt. So, he began to pray. He prayed that God would allow him to do something about Jerusalem.

God answered his prayer. The king gave Nehemiah permission to return and gave him a voucher to purchase everything he would need to make the necessary repairs to the walls of Jerusalem so as to not leave them vulnerable to being raided or attacked by marauders or enemies. When he got there, he took three days to simply survey the damage and come up with a plan to do the work.

Now, here is where it gets good. He finally met with the leaders in Jerusalem and said, "… You see the distress that we are in, how Jerusalem lies in waste, and its gates are burned with fire. Come, let us build the wall of Jerusalem…" (Nehemiah 2:17, NKJV).

Nehemiah had to state the obvious…you are living in despair! They had lived in desolation so long that they had grown used to it and accepted it as their lifestyle, as normal. Nehemiah came in with a fresh pair of eyes and saw what could be done and rallied the people to rebuild.

We all need "Nehemiahs" in our lives. We need people to help us see things for what they really are. However, don't wait for someone to magically show up. Instead invite people to speak truth into your life. Choose a few trustworthy people and give them permission to tell you when you "are living in despair." Find some trustworthy sober supports, an accountability partner and possibly the most important if you have an addiction, get a sponsor. When you feel discouraged in the future, the sponsor will be a friend who lifts you up and restores your hope.

Jeremiah gave hope to the citizens of Jerusalem, and this is a stirring message of hope and determination from which we can all learn and grow. So many times, we live our lives in desolation and despair. We come to accept it as our lot in life and take it as normal. Living in addiction is not normal or healthy! The wreckage and the desolation left in the wake of our addictions is not the way it needs to be. God has better plans for us. His eyes see what can be done. He is not finished with you. His work is not done. He wants to rebuild us! Will you begin the process of allowing him to rebuild you? He will provide us with hope when our life seems wasted, shattered and ruined.

As a clinical psychologist, I (Jared) know that one of the most important curative factors involved in the psychotherapeutic process is the instillation of hope. According to the research, providing distressed, despairing, despondent clients a sense of hope is what inspires and injects healing. Hope heals our hurting hearts.

Yet when we are in the midst of our deepest pain and the subsequent recurring and addictive ways we attempt to medicate it, sometimes the only thing we can muster up hope for is the next drink, fix, high or rush. It is precisely in these dark and desperate places that the psalmist asks us rhetorically: "Why are you in despair, O my soul? And why have you become restless and disturbed within me? Hope in God and wait expectantly for Him..." (Psalm 42:5, AMP).

This Biblical concept of hope is not some unrealistic, Pollyanna-ish "pie in the sky in the sweet bye and bye" type of religious denial system. This rock solid sense of hopeful expectation is grounded firmly on the promises within the unchanging Word of God. Throughout scripture we are comforted by the Father's unfailing loving assurance that He has a hope and a future plan for our lives no matter our current state of temporary painful, scary or uncertain circumstances (Jeremiah 29:11, Proverbs 23:18, Isaiah 40:31, Romans 15:4, 1 Corinthians 15:19). "We have this hope as an anchor for the soul, firm and secure..." (Hebrews 6:19, NIV), so "Let us seize and hold tightly the confessions of our hope without wavering, for He who promised is reliable and trustworthy and faithful to His Word" Hebrews 10:23, AMP).

As a senior in medical school, I (Paul) was very stressed out. We had people's lives in our hands and worked very long hours. When I learned to deliver babies, we showed up at 6 a.m. and worked 36 straight hours until 6 p.m. the next day with no sleep. Then we got twelve hours off and repeated the cycle. They wanted to break us in to a schedule we might be expected at times to experience when we would have emergencies in the future. I remember getting so discouraged that I raised my books over my head and was ready to throw them on the floor and quit medical school.

But my friend, Frank Minirth, gave me hope. He reminded me that we only had a few months to go to finish medical school, and that our residencies would not be as difficult, and then we would be free to determine what field of medicine to go into and practice and set our own hours and determine what responsibilities we could handle. The rest of our lives would be what we had dreamed of since our teen years, but we would have to suffer for three more months.

He said that if we had to wade in mud for the next three months it would still be worth it for the privilege of helping people in the medical specialty of our choice for the rest of our lives, as God had called us to do. I put my books back by my side and marched on to our next class, then back to the bedsides to deliver more babies, which was very exciting anyway. Who can you give hope and encouragement to today? Pray for an opportunity and do it.

Daily Surrender and Reflection

Please spend a few moments reflecting on how you have at times become comfortable in your sickness and sin. How can you avoid complacency in your spiritual walk and recovery? Do you have any "Nehemiahs" in your life? If so who are they? If not, who can you ask? What are the things for which you need the Father to give you hope?

_____

_____

_____

_____

_____

_____

_____

_____

_____

_____

_____

_____

_____

_____

DAY TEN

Word of the Day: *Wisdom*

Scripture: "Walk with the wise and become wise; associate with fools and get in trouble." (Proverbs 13:20, NLT)

Quote: "Remember that we deal with alcohol, cunning, baffling, powerful! Without help it is too much for us. But there is One who has all power that One is God. May you find Him now!" (Alcoholics Anonymous, 1st. Edition)

Be Wise in Your Recovery

Proverbs has a lot of profound things to say about the perils of alcohol; the perils with which we are all too familiar. One of the most striking of these is found in Proverbs 20:1: "Wine is a mocker, strong drink a brawler; and whoever is led astray by it is not wise" (ESV). The Message version puts it even more graphically: "Wine makes you mean, beer makes you quarrelsome--a staggering drunk is not much fun."

On the surface of this verse, there is practical instruction. Have you ever been under the influence of alcohol and said or did something stupid? In that sense, alcohol mocks us. Have you ever been or seen an angry drunk? In that sense, strong drink is a brawler. Practical and to the point.

What is said next takes the struggle against addiction and alcoholism to the core issue. This is something the founders of AA understood deeply. The core issue is a conflict of kingdoms. The passage says, "and whoever is led astray by it is not wise."

We tend to interpret this to mean, "whoever is led astray by it is not smart," but that is not the true meaning. In the Bible, to be wise is much more than knowing something. It is also to apply that knowledge, and in this case, it is applying God's Word. The wise person knows God's Word and applies God's Word, therefore living as though God is relevant in his life.

To be unwise, then, is to live as though God is not relevant in our lives; to arrogantly try to live as though God is not there. What is the opposite of being wise? It is to be a fool. "The fool says in his heart, 'there is no God'" (Psalm 14:1, (NIV))..

Many say we believe in God, but we live as if there is no God. Charles Spurgeon called this being a practical atheist--someone who for all practical purposes lives life as if there is no God. They live for their own hedonistic desires and selfish needs. So we see at the heart and core of our struggle is a kingdom conflict: God's Kingdom or our kingdom. That is why the founders of AA, Dr. Bob and Bill W. saw the need for us all to submit our lives and wills over to God. That is why applying the 12 steps to our lives is really about living as though God is very relevant in our lives. Therein lies the strength and the power. His power.

Years ago I (Paul) treated a movie star who was rich, famous, successful, but suicidally depressed because she was going through her seventh divorce. She wanted to do what was right, and was a believer, but lacked wisdom and insight. She married seven abusive alcoholics in a row, not knowing that any of them were alcoholics until after the wedding vows had been said all seven times. They all ran around on her as well, and beat her up if she complained about it. She thought all of them were nice when she dated them. But she had blinders on.

The first day I met her and did my one hour work up, instead of asking her about her childhood, I told her what I thought it must have been like. I told her that her dad had probably been an alcoholic, and that he probably beat up on Alice's (not her real name) mother, and that he had been unfaithful, and that he probably even sexually abused Alice growing up. Alice was shocked that I had guessed all of this correctly and asked me how I did that. I told her about codependency, and how that meant that she had an unconscious need to repeat her childhood. She had a need to fix her childhood. She wanted the genuine love of her father and never received it. She was bitter toward him and wanted vengeance as well. She saw herself as a perpetual victim. When she was single and dated different men, she was bored whenever she dated a really nice and godly man.

The men she married acted nice, but she could unconsciously sense the truth about them—that they were secretly much like her father. So she "fell in love" with each of them and married them to try to fix her childhood and finally get the love of a father substitute. She enabled each of them, letting them get away with their abuse and alcoholism until she finally divorced each one at her giving up point in each marriage. But she was blind to all of this. In therapy in our Day Program for seven hours a day for the next three weeks, she gained insight and wisdom into how our unconscious tricks us into making the same foolish mistakes over and over again.

By gaining wisdom and insight, she was able to grieve her childhood losses and quit trying to fix them by being addicted to alcoholics who were also abusive and unfaithful. She got over her depression and never married or even dated an abusive man after that. She got wisdom and applied it.

The Bible declares wisdom to be the most valuable and precious commodity we can possess. The wisest man who ever lived, King Solomon (who was so wise because God gave him that wisdom at his request--see 1 Kings 4:29-34) told us that "Wisdom is supreme; therefore get wisdom. Though it cost all you have, get understanding" (Proverbs 4:7, NIV). You may ask, "how do I acquire wisdom, insight and understanding?" James 1:5 reveals the answer: "If any of you lacks wisdom, you should ask God, who gives generously to all without finding fault, and it will be given to you" (NIV).

David prayed at the end of Psalm 139 for God to reveal to David his own innermost thoughts, so David could learn to walk in a way that was pleasing to God. Pray for wisdom into your own unconscious dynamics today, so you and God can take control of your life instead of allowing your unconscious sinful nature and Satan rule your life without you even recognizing it.

Live today as though God is relevant in your life, for the rest of your life, and for your recovery. That is supreme wisdom!

Daily Surrender and Reflection

Now please think this through, are you wise? Do you ask for wisdom? In what areas would you like to become more wise? Ask someone you trust how you need to grow in wisdom. Then spend a few moments reflecting on which areas of your life you could live more wisely:

_____

_____

_____

_____

_____

_____

_____

_____

_____

_____

_____

_____

_____

_____

DAY ELEVEN

Word: *Silence*

Scripture: "For God alone, O my soul, wait in silence, for my hope is from him." (Psalm 62:5, ESV)

Quote: "We should fix ourselves firmly in the presence of God by conversing all the time with him... we should feed our soul with a lofty conception of God and from that derive great joy in being his. We should put life in our faith. We should give ourselves utterly to God in pure abandonment, in temporal and spiritual matters alike, and find contentment in the doing of his will, whether he takes us through sufferings or consolations. " (Brother Lawrence)

Shutting Off The Noise

I (Paul) read my Bible and pray almost every day of my life, and have for over sixty years now. But I often forget to be silent and just be patiently quiet for a while and listen for the Lord to speak to me—to guide me or give me a new insight. I pray for things and pray for people but often forget to listen. Prayer should be a two way conversation. Oh, I never hear God's voice out loud! I would take medication to make those voices go away if I heard that kind of voice! But I hear God's "still, small voice"—as the Bible calls it (1 Kings 19:12)—speaking from his Spirit to my own spirit.

Sometimes, when under a lot of stress, I will go to a gym nearby and go to the hot tub at an hour in the early morning or late at night when nobody else is there, and just float on my back, looking up toward God.

The smoke rising from the hot water reminds me of how our prayers are lifted up to God and he considers it like pleasant incense in his nostrils. Floating on my back reminds me of my dependence on God to lift me up. And I quit talking to God after a while, and just float there and listen for God to speak to me—and he does speak to me.

In our culture today, we get very busy and even our private lives stay busy with social media and other activities. Facebook, Twitter, Pinterest, SnapChat, Linkedin, Radio, Cellphone, Email… the list goes on and on. It seems our world has become inundated with noise. And it's really tough to be able to hear a still small voice amid all the clatter, clanging and cacophony of noise.

The other day I (Phil) was with my family at a four year old's birthday party. In the midst of all the festivities between the games, the cake and presents, I took a couple phone calls, and I troubleshot some problems at the office with an email, I also tweeted a post or two and read a couple of status updates. Then, standing in the middle of this child's birthday party, I felt some emotions welling up inside of me. So I put my phone down.

A little overwhelmed, I sat down and felt this amazing range of emotions from anxiety to pure elated joy and everything in between. I turned to my wife and said "Hon, I don't understand, I just feel overwhelmed right now." As I sat and tried to quiet myself in the midst of the distractions, I heard the music playing in the background for the first time all day. It was the song that was playing as my beautiful bride was walking down the aisle so many years before. The song had brought up inside me all of the emotions from my wedding day, but I was so distracted with the "noise", I couldn't hear them.

In times like these, I have to remember what The LORD said in 1 Kings 19:11-13. The LORD said, "Go out and stand on the mountain in the presence of the LORD, for the LORD is about to pass by." Then a great and powerful wind tore the mountains apart and shattered the rocks before the LORD, but the LORD was not in the wind. After the wind there was an earthquake, but the LORD was not in the earthquake. After the earthquake came a fire, but the LORD was not in the fire. And after the fire came a gentle whisper" (NIV).

A whisper is a very intimate and powerful form of communication. Someone whispers something to us that is personal, privileged and private.

But in order to clearly perceive that message, we must focus our full attention onto the messenger and their communication to us. It's hard to hear a whisper when we are surrounded by chaos, contentiousness and calamity.

There are a lot of great things in our noisy and distracting world that fight for our attention. Sometimes we will need to say no to good things to receive the best. Other times, the distractions and diversions which clamor for our attention are things which are or can become addictive and life controlling. This journey of recovery demands that we shut off the external and extraneous noise and listen for God's direction. Will you join me in shutting off the noise, and listening for the still, small voice of God, our Father's intimate whisper?

Daily Surrender and Reflection

Spend a few minutes reflecting on the noise and distractions in your life. What noise needs to be shut off? What changes can you make in your life to facilitate reducing the distractions in your life? Spend a few moments in silence, and allow yourself to listen for God's still small voice. What do you feel like God is trying to tell you when you listen to him in silence, patiently? Answer these questions and journal about this experience.

_____

_____

_____

_____

_____

_____

_____

_____

_____

_____

_____

_____

_____

_____

DAY TWELVE

Word of the Day: *Humility*

Scripture: "He heals the brokenhearted and bandages their wounds. He counts the stars and calls them all by name. How great is our Lord! His power is absolute! His understanding is beyond comprehension! The Lord supports the humble, but he brings the wicked down into the dust." (Psalm 147:3-6, NLT)

Quote: "…we had to quit playing God. It didn't work. Next, we decided that hereafter in this drama of life, God was going to be our Director. He is the Principal; we are His agents. He is the Father and we are His children. Most good ideas are simple, and this concept was the keystone of the new and triumphant arch through which we passed to freedom." (Alcoholics Anonymous Big Book, p.62)

There Is A God And I Am Not Him

At times all of us – especially those of us with addictive tendencies or full blown addictions – believe that we are the protagonist (the leading character) and have been cast in the "star" role in the story of our life. However, the truth is that we are at best a supporting character in a much more majestic tale. The story is simply not ours. It is God's story. It's not a story about you; it's a story about him. God is the protagonist, the author, the producer, the director and the creator. He is the Great I Am, the Alpha and Omega, and God allows us to play a part in his love story.

The actor Robert Prosky, playing the role of Father Cavanaugh in the movie Rudy, said it best, "Son, in 35 years of religious study, I have only come up with two hard incontrovertible facts: there is a God, and I'm not him."

God deeply loves us, however, we are not his equals. He is God and we are His, not the other way around. When I (Phil) reflect on my supporting role in this broken journey of life, I haven't always been the best decision maker. In fact, it is pretty clear that my decisions do not typically reflect the decisions of an all knowing deity. I'm wrong so very often. Reminiscing I can't help but cringe at some of the amazingly immature and self-centered requests I have laid before God.

With every year that passes, I notice more and more my prayers changing. I now thank God for not answering many of my past passion filled requests. I thank God for being God and I thank him that I am not. I now find myself praying "Not my will, but yours be done," praying that God will have his way with me and teach me what he wants. This concept offers me great support as I begin to recognize that "there is a God, and I'm not him."

Actually, the very essence of our sin nature is to selfishly and pridefully try to "be as God." Ever since Genesis chapter 3 (the account of the Fall of man), we have wanted to be in charge. I (Jared) know that for me, every time I want to be in charge and want what I want, when I want it, how I want it, because I want it, the Holy Spirit has to remind me that I am in fact, not the emperor potentate of the universe.

That reassurance always comforts and blesses me. It's a pretty tough job to be in control of the whole world, and there is only one who has the ability, qualifications and experience to do it! The overwhelming arrogance of my temptation to pride is not only an affront to the LORD (boss) of the (His) entire world, it always harms me and others in my world as well.

I (Paul) remember two special occasions in my life where God had to supernaturally humble me. When the Soviet Empire fell, and Boris Yeltsin, a good man, became the first President of the new Russian Federation in 1991, he allowed Christian missionaries to come into Russia with total freedom to spread the gospel. This is no longer the way things are in Russia.

I had the privilege of going there for a missions trip and saw God work through our team in a truly supernatural way. I stood in Red Square with a

Coke in my hand, toasting the new Russian soldiers, yelling out, "Yeltsin, Yeltsin." I got to train psychiatrists and psychologists about Christian psychology in Moscow. Then my team went to St. Petersburg where I had the privilege to teach about a hundred psychology graduate students about Christian psychology for a whole week at the university there, with about half of them becoming Christians by the end of the week.

I taught an older, established psychologist in the area who was a devout atheist and did not want to know anything about God but wanted to know what techniques we used at the Meier Clinics in America. In fact, when I gave her a Russian Bible, she practically threw it down on the next chair, saying she did not want it. I asked her if I could pretend like she was a new patient of mine and do a work up on her. I knew immediately that since she was so hostile toward the idea of a Supreme Being, she was probably angry at an absent father in her own life. She also looked sad to me, and she smoked nonstop.

So just by observing her body language and first few words, I asked her if her father was gone most of the time growing up. She looked surprised that I guessed that and said that he had been a sailor and was gone six months at a time when she was growing up and she resented not having a father to experience. Most of us end up marrying someone similar to our own parent of the opposite sex, so I asked her if she married someone to whom she never got to feel connected, who was also distant like her father had been. At that point she began to cry and said she had married someone like that and had recently gone through a divorce.

Most people who smoke too much also drink too much, so I asked her if she had a drinking problem and she said she did drink too much. Then she asked my friend Doug and I a spiritual question, and Doug started quoting her a passage of scripture that obvious was starting to impact her spiritually. But Doug couldn't remember how the passage ended and could not remember where the passage was found. I couldn't either, even though I had also memorized that passage in the past.

But we had hired a Russian college kid to be our interpreter, and he grabbed the Russian Bible she had discarded and opened it at random and finished reading the passage that Doug had begun to quote to her. Then, realizing what he had just done, he dropped the Bible and trembled and asked us how he had just done that? I told him and her that God had enabled him to do that because He loved them both. They both became believers.

I went to bed that night giving myself way too much credit for all the amazing things that had taken place that week, and fell asleep thinking how lucky God was to have me as a Christian Psychiatrist doing all these wonderful things for Him. I immediately had a dream where all my major sins from early childhood one were flashed before my eyes, one at a time, and I woke up weeping and apologizing to God for being so prideful. The Holy Spirit lovingly made me feel close and feel forgiven but reminded me that God uses the foolish things of this world to confound the wise. I fell asleep in peace, much more humble. I didn't tell anybody about the dream. The next morning the team leader started our devotions after breakfast, and said he changed the verse he was going to speak on because of a dream he had last night. The verse he spoke on was I Corinthians 1:27, about how God uses the foolish things of the world to confound the wise. It was an affirmation to me that God was serious in wanting me to be more humble, so I shared my dream experience also at that time.

Two years later I was able to get into Cuba, rather miraculously since American tourists were not allowed to go there at the time. I got to teach Christian psychology to about 1000 medical doctors in Havana and Cienfuegos, Cuba, and many became believers. I even got to teach some of Castro's cabinet officials. They had a spy assigned to me to be sure I said nothing negative about Fidel Castro. We got to speak to large crowds of children for whom we did clown shows first. About 700 Cubans became Christians at our meetings that week.

On the last day, I fell asleep very proud of myself again, just like I had two years earlier in Russia, telling God how lucky He was to have me. I had the same dream, with my major sins flashing before my eyes, with new ones added from the previous two years, and again woke up crying and apologizing to God. The Holy Spirit comforted me again, showing me the verse about how God's strength is used through us the more we realize how weak we are without him. Again, I told nobody about my dream. The team leader led our devotions the next morning after breakfast. Again, he said he had changed his mind about what to share based on a dream he had the night before. He shared II Corinthians 12:9, about how God's strength is made perfect in our weakness.

Daily Surrender and Reflection

Have you tried to be God in your own life? Have you tried to arrogantly inform God on how things should be done? Have you thought you knew better than God? Please spend a few moments reflecting on these questions. What areas in your life do you need to humble yourself before God and surrender your will? Use the below space to journal about your thoughts in this regard:

_____

_____

_____

_____

_____

_____

_____

_____

_____

_____

_____

_____

_____

DAY THIRTEEN

Word of the Day: *Truth*

Scripture: "...If you hold to my teaching, you are really my disciples. Then you will know the truth, and the truth will set you free," John 31-32, NIV)

Quote: "There are two ways to be fooled. One is to believe what isn't true; the other is to refuse to believe what is true." (Søren Kierkegaard)

Replacing Lies with the Truth of God

Each of us have an internal "voice" or internal dialogue in our heads. This is often referred to as self-talk. Our self-talk can be positive or negative. Effective counseling often begins with helping a person to identify the negative self-talk and replace those thoughts with positive ones. At its heart, this is a solidly Christian and very effective technique. We as Christians believe that knowing and internalizing the Truth will set us free.

According to the Mayo Clinic, people who experience positive self-talk "...live healthier lifestyles – they get more physical activity, follow a healthier diet, and have reduced rates of smoking and alcohol consumption." We actually become what we think about.

Many of us have false beliefs about ourselves. Some of us feel unlovable, incapable, and at times unworthy. However, simply telling ourselves positive things sometimes falls short. We believe the Truth found in the scriptures of the Bible will never fall short. The Scriptures are more than just words on a page. They are the living word of God. Speaking the truth of scripture into our lives can transform us.

Let's practice replacing the lies (negative self-talk) with the Truth (The Word of God). For instance, you're struggling with the lie that you are unlovable lets replace that thought with Isaiah 43:4 "You are precious and honored in My sight, and I love you" [version?]. God loves you. If the God of the universe loves you, you are certainly lovable.

Here are just a few more examples of this transformational technique:

Lie: "I am a failure. I can't do anything right."
Truth: Philippians 4:13 — "I can do all things through Christ who strengthens me" (NKJV).

Lie: "I am alone."
Truth: Hebrews. 13:5 — "...God has said, 'never will I leave you; never will I forsake you'" (NIV).

Lie: "I am worthless, ugly, etc."
Truth: Ephesians. 2:10 — "For we are God's masterpiece. He has created us anew in Christ Jesus" [version?].

Lie: "I've done too many evil things. I could never be forgiven."
Truth: Hebrews 8:12 "For I will forgive their wickedness and will remember their sins no more) (NIV).

Lie: "I am only deserving of judgment because my guilt is so severe."
Truth: Romans 8:1 "Therefore, there is now no condemnation for those who are in Christ Jesus" (NIV).

This is an especially powerful verse when you look at it in context of the chapter that comes before that verse, chapter seven of Romans. In chapter seven, the Apostle Paul admits that, even though he strives to be a godly person, he sometimes does things he should not do, and he sometimes does not do the things he knows he should do. He tells how painful that is when he fails in those regards, saying "Woe is me." But he concludes with the promise of God's undeserved, unchanging and unconditional grace in Romans 8:1, "Therefore, there is now NO CONDEMNATION...." (emphasis added).

God's goal is not to condemn us for our failures, but to show us that He does not condemn us for being human, but rather wants us to learn from our mistakes and grow from them. The world, or legalistic Christians, may call us a failure. But God says the truth is that there is no condemnation for us. This principle is also emphasized in the next sentence after perhaps the most famous verse in the Bible (John 3:16). Jesus explained that "God did not send his Son into the world to condemn the world, but to save the world through him (John 3:17, NIV). Our guilt was fully paid for at the cross of Calvary. Jesus' atonement for our sin is the essence of the Good News!

Therefore, we live in God's grace and forgiveness. What does God call a person who fails seven times in a row but keeps on getting back up and trying again to surrender to God and live for him? The world calls him an utter failure. But, in Proverbs 24:16, God calls him "a righteous man." We are not righteous due to our own actions but because of the sacrificial life, death and resurrection of Jesus Christ.

God's Truth, applied with love and wisdom, will never return void (Isaiah 53:9). Practice today replacing the lies with the truth of God.

Daily Surrender and Reflection

What lies or negative self-talk have you believed about yourself? Spend a few moments reflecting on the lies. List each lie in the space provided. Please spend a few moments reflecting on the concept of truth. What are some truths that the scriptures say about you? Spend a few moments reflecting of these truths. Remember God wants the truth to set you free.

_____

_____

_____

_____

_____

_____

_____

_____

_____

_____

_____

_____

_____

_____

DAY FOURTEEN

Word of the Day: *Unlikely*

Scripture: "But God had mercy on me so that Christ Jesus could use me as a prime example of his great patience with even the worst sinners. Then others will realize that they, too, can believe in him and receive eternal life." (1 Timothy 1:16, NLT)

Quote: "God isn't looking for perfect people to use. He is looking to use imperfect people whom he makes perfect through Jesus." (Pastor James Exline)

God Uses Unlikely People

Are you an "unlikely"? If you have a "checkered past", if you've done things you've been ashamed of, then congratulations, you are an "unlikely" and God wants to use you! You may have heard that God has plans for you, that God wants to use you, but then you look at yourself, your past, and begin to develop a laundry list of reasons why God wouldn't use you. You begin to disqualify yourself.

It can be easy to look at the "spiritual greats" and think of course God would use them-- just look at what they accomplished! This, however, is not an accurate portrait of those "spiritual greats." This lens leaves out the fact that they were imperfect people being used by a perfect God to accomplish his perfect will and perfect plan. The perfect part of the equation comes from God—not the person God is using—and not from you!

In Matthew 5:48 and other places, the Bible implies that we, as believers, should "be perfect." But the English language does not give justice in these passages to what God's Word is actually saying in the original languages. The Greek words used in these New Testament passages is always either "artios" or "telios," both of which mean to be MATURE, or fully developed, not perfect. In fact, the Bible says in many other places, including I John chapter one, that we cannot be perfect, and that if anyone says he is perfect, he is a liar. Perfection comes in heaven, not on earth.

Let's look at some imperfect people God has used; even a partial list is very interesting. God used a person who ordered the persecution and murder of Christians, (the Apostle Paul, formerly known as Saul) to write over half of the New Testament and lead countless numbers of people to a relationship with Christ. He used a murderer and a stutterer (Moses) to lead his people out of slavery to freedom. He used a little shepherd boy (about whom his father called him the "least" of his family), to defeat a giant and later this little David became king of God's people. David then went on to commit adultery, murder and the list goes on. Peter, the leader of the early church, denied knowing Jesus. That's right, the guy God later used to establish the church claimed on three separate occasions that he did not even know Jesus!

In fact, none of the "heroes of the faith" were anywhere near perfect, righteous or holy. They were all flawed, failed, fallen humans. The Bible never sugarcoats or whitewashes either sin or sinners. Scriptural characters are always accurately portrayed in all their inglorious dysfunctions, inconsistencies, struggles and sinfulness.

Take some time to carefully investigate the personalities and their life histories listed in the Old Testament "hall of fame" in Hebrews chapter 11. These ancients were all "commended for their faith" (verse 2, NIV) but let's look closely at their infamous if not downright notorious pasts. The list includes people who were drunks, liars, thieves, adulterers, murders, prostitutes, spoiled brats, cowards, outcasts and misfits.

Pretty motley crew huh? Do you still think you are an "unlikely?" But those tabloid headline-like facts about these patriarch's lives are not what they are remembered or known for. These "unlikely" servants of God are actually among the most highly revered Bible characters--not because of their sinful and sordid pasts, but because they were commended for their faith in and submission to God.

You may have been enslaved to active alcoholism and addiction for years, and along the way did things which many would think had disqualified you from being used by God. You may be thinking there is no way God would ever use you, after all, just look at the long list of disqualifications!

You have a list of disqualifications, things that you believe are preventing you from being used by God. You look at your past, and come to the conclusion that "God will never use me." "You don't understand," you might say. "I've done..." the list goes on and on. From looking at that list from a human perspective, you may be justified in thinking that God will never use you.

The good news, however, is that God does not look at you or your past from a human perspective. He looks at it through the redeeming, saving, and salvaging eyes of perfect love, through the eyes of a savior who died for you to become the very righteousness of God!

2 Corinthians 5:21 says, "For our sake he (God) made him (Jesus) to be sin who knew no sin, so that in him we might become the righteousness of God" (NIV). When God the Father looks at you, he sees you clothed in the robe of the perfect Jesus, in a robe of righteousness, and declares you perfect because of what Jesus did for you when you received Him, not based on what you have done or not done in your life.

God isn't looking for perfect people to use. He is looking to use imperfect people whom he makes perfect (mature) through Jesus. So you're not perfect, congratulations, you qualify! That's where the good news comes in for you. If you are imperfect, if you have a "checkered past," and if you are willing to allow God to use you to accomplish his plans through you, then you qualify! God wants to use you!

Daily Surrender and Reflection

Are you an unlikely? Have you ever felt disqualified to be used by God? Have you thought you couldn't be forgiven for what you've done? Spend a few moments journaling about these thoughts and reflecting on the fact that God desires to use you and has great plans for you.

_____

_____

_____

_____

_____

_____

_____

_____

_____

_____

_____

_____

_____

_____

_____

_____

DAY FIFTEEN

Word of the Day: *Speaking*

Scripture: "The tongue has the power of life and death..." (Proverbs 18:21, NIV)

Quote: "Remember that the tongue speaks only what is in the heart." (Theodore Epp)

Words Matter

"With the tongue we praise our Lord and Father, and with it we curse human beings, who have been made in God's likeness. Out of the same mouth come praise and cursing. My brothers and sisters, this should not be. Can both fresh water and salt water flow from the same spring? My brothers and sisters, can a fig tree bear olives, or a grapevine bear figs? Neither can a salt spring produce fresh water" (James 3:9-12, (NIV).

Curse noun 1. the expression of a wish that misfortune, evil, doom, etc., befall a person, group, etc.; a profane oath; curse word.

As a young boy I (Phil) remember my grandmother overhearing me saying some very vulgar statements about a young girl and my grandma looked me in the eye and said "You kiss me with that mouth?" You may have received a similar correction as a child, "you kiss your mother with that mouth?" James is saying a kindred statement in the above scripture. You praise God with that mouth?

Follow James' logic here for a moment. We claim to have a relationship with God as our Lord and Father. Out of one side of our mouth we praise

God and then curse our neighbors, our family, even ourselves out of that same mouth. We have a problem.

God is great, God is powerful, God is love and God is God. When we curse others or even ourselves, when we say that person is a jerk, or I'm an idiot, I'm worthless, etc., the one we curse is made in the likeness of and is a reflection of the Lord and Father.

"So God created man in his own image, in the image of God He created him; male and female He created them" (Gen 1:27 ESV). We have the unique honor of being God's image bearers. Therefore, to treat people with contempt, to treat ourselves like the stuff we scrape off the bottom of our shoes, is to treat God's own image with contempt.

I deeply love my children. My son Judah has a special place in my heart. Let us imagine for a moment you walk up to me and tell me how much you love me, respect me and even admire me. You lay it on pretty thick. Then I see you moments latter walking up to my son Judah and you begin to berate him, yell at him and tell him he is a good for nothing worthless kid. Would I think you still loved me? Or respected me? Of course not. But this is what we do to God every day when we demean or disrespect one of His kids.

"The tongue has the power of life and death..." (Proverbs 18:21, NIV). This little muscle, the tongue, is powerful. There was a season in my life where I had been so broken that all it took was a few words to destroy any fiber of hope I had. I remember contemplating taking my life, because of some words someone had spoken. Likewise I can tell you that in some of my darkest moments just a few words of encouragement have rescued me from that brink and brought me back to life. Remember that words are powerful and choose today to speak life into yourself and those around you.

When I (Paul) was a twelve year old boy, I was planning on growing up and becoming a carpenter, like my dad, and maybe even working with him some day. There is nothing wrong with those dreams. God calls many to become carpenters. Jesus' own dad, Joseph, was a carpenter. But a very elderly widow in our church, Mrs. Arnold, came up to me after a church service and surprised me by laying both of her hands on my shoulders and told me, "Paul, I am praying for you every day, and I believe God is going to use you in a very special way to bring many people to Him." I was surprised, but thanked her and pondered those words and still do ponder them nearly sixty years later. I wondered as a youth how I could fulfill that prediction she made.

By age 16 I felt called by God to become a Christian physician and to use that as a platform to further the cause of Christ. Several million people have come to Christ over the decades as a result of various Meier Clinic ministries, radio, TV, books, international training, and spin off ministries that we started, including Women of Faith, an enormous ministry that was created by the Minirth-Meier New Life Clinics a couple decades ago. Mrs. Arnold's few positive words changed my life, and the destinies of many others.

Words are very impactful indeed. For good or for evil. Again, wise King Solomon frequently guides us about our speech throughout the book of Proverbs. A few of these dozens of life-giving principles include: "When there are many words, transgression and offense are unavoidable, but he who controls his lips and keeps thoughtful silence is wise" (10:19, AMP), "The one who has knowledge uses words with restraint, and whoever has understanding is even tempered. Even fools are thought wise if they keep silent, and discerning if they hold their tongue" (17:27-28, NIV), and "Watch your words and hold your tongue; you'll save yourself a lot of grief" (21:23, MSG).

Jesus taught us that whatever is inside our heart is what is going to spill out whenever we're bumped (Luke 6:45). That's why the Apostle Paul later advised us to "Let your speech always be gracious, seasoned with salt, so that you may know how you ought to answer each person" (Colossians 4:6, ESV). What we say, and perhaps more importantly how we say it (i.e., tone of voice, nonverbal expressions, etc.), can literally make or break our relationships, determine the course of our futures and result in others and ourselves being either blessed or cursed.

Daily Surrender and Reflection

Please spend a few moments reflecting on your tongue. How have you spoken life and how have you spoken death? Can you think of a few ways you could speak life into someone today? How can you honor God with your words today? Use the below space to answer these questions and to journal about how you could improve how you can use the powerful tool of words.

_____

_____

_____

_____

_____

_____

_____

_____

_____

_____

_____

_____

_____

DAY SIXTEEN:

Word of the Day: *Sex*

Scripture: "It is God's will that you should be sanctified: that you should avoid sexual immorality; that each of you should learn to control your own body in a way that is holy and honorable, not in passionate lust like the pagans, who do not know God." (1 Thessalonians 4:3-5, NIV)

Quote: "By trying to grab fulfillment everywhere, we find it nowhere." – (Elisabeth Elliot)

The Gift of Sex

Sex was not created on some sleazy adult website. Sex, our sex drive, and sexual pleasure were created by the Creator himself. Our sexual life is of great concern to God. Some of us are rebels. We're addicts, we don't like people telling us what to do. We want to live life on our own terms. We might not like it, we might rebel against his ownership, but we still are God's. He made you, he bought you at a price and has an absolute right to tell you what is good for you.

The Bible states that your body is not your own: "Do you not know that your body is the temple of the Holy Spirit, within you, which you have from God? You are not your own; you were bought with a price. So glorify God in your body" (I Corinthians 6:19-20, [version?]). Oh, what an offensive word to our sexually liberated, sexually free, I'm my own, nobody is going to tell me what to do, culture.

The body in which you dwell is not yours to do with simply as you please. God has bought your body, Jesus bought your body with the whip marks across his back and the nails in his hands and feet. God bought you from your bondage with the payment of his own Son, and now our bodies should serve one all-encompassing purpose: "Glorify God in your body."

As Paul said in Romans 6:12–14, "Let not sin therefore reign in your mortal bodies to make you obey their passions. Do not yield yourselves to sin as instruments of wickedness, but yield yourselves to God as people who have been brought from death to life, and your bodily parts to God as instruments of righteousness. For sin will have no dominion over you, for you are not under law but under grace" ([version]).

God has brought you from death to life. God is concerned about what you do with your body. He created your body, he bought it, he owns it, he indwells within you, and what you do with it demonstrates to the world who your Lord is.

I (Phil) have this slightly deformed decades old stuffed teddy bear. I made this bear when I was young as a gift for my Grandmother. I spent hours cutting and stitching this bear together. I loved my Grandmother. I was her Baby Lamb, I was her favorite and she adored me. When my Grandmother passed a few years back, she had kidney failure, and for weeks before she died, she had slowly been giving away all her belongings. In fact, her room was pretty empty towards the end.

But sitting on her shelf where she could see it, up to the point of her death, was this deformed little bear. She protected this bear. The great grandkids would come over and run around her room, but she refused to let them play with the bear. Not because it is a beautiful bear (even though, I did a pretty good job). It was obvious to all that she loved and cherished the bear not because of the bear, but because she adored the one who created and gave her the bear.

Sex is a blessing. A great gift that should be cherished. But are you cherishing the gift more than the gift giver. You see how you value the gift exposes how you feel about the one who gave you the gift. How you treat your body, your sexual life, reveals how you truly feel about the one who gave you the gift of sexuality. The scriptures say that we are God's masterpiece. That when we are reborn in Jesus Christ we are God's Magnum Opus. Is the way you are treating your body, your sexuality, telling God that you cherish Him, that you love Him? Or are you sending a different message to Him and the world around you?

However, when we struggle with sexual addiction or have deep pain in the private realm of our sexuality, it may seem like God's grand, glorious gift of sex is more like a demonic, devastating damnation. To persons who have been wounded, exploited victimized and/or assaulted in the most intimate and vulnerable areas of their humanity, sex can be one of the cruelest curses in all of creation. Whether it be from childhood sexual trauma (research suggests approximately one in three girls and one in four to six boys are molested in America), the betrayal of infidelity, the widespread scourge of pornography, painful promiscuous or unmarried relationships, or the ravages of a dysfunctional and unhealthy marriage, sexual hurts are horrible.

I (Jared) have treated thousands of survivors of childhood sexual abuse, victims of assault, troubled marriages and addicts over the years, and I want to tell you dear sister or brother, even though you don't dare allow yourself to believe it, there is help, hope and healing for your horrible hurts. Find a good, well-qualified and experienced Christian therapist who will walk with you through the journey of tragedy of harmfulness to the triumph of sexual wholeness.

The reality is that sex can be more heavenly glorious in God's perfect design in a healthy marriage or more horribly grotesque than anything else in all of creation. To borrow metaphors from classic literature, it can be the best of times or the worst of times, agony or ecstasy.

When I (Paul) was in medical school, I remember when one of our professors was teaching us about human sexuality. He said that all humans are tempted to have sex with people other than our mate from time to time. He said if anyone never has any sexual temptations, he should go to the emergency room quick because he is either sick or dead. So we should not condemn ourselves for being normal humans with temptations. The Bible says that Jesus was tempted in all ways just like we are, but without sin.

Our brief, momentary temptations become a sin when we dwell on them and amplify them and, worst of all, when we act out on them. Job, one of the godliest men who ever lived, struggled with sexual temptations, but he said that he came to a point where he made a vow with his eyes to not look on women with lust. We need to see members of the opposite sex as sons and daughters of God and as human eternal souls, not just in terms of their body parts or how good it might temporarily feel to use that person sexually, bringing pain to yourself and that other person later.

Daily Surrender and Reflection

Please spend a few moments reflecting on the message your sexual life has been sending to God and others. Are your choices telling God you cherish Him above your feelings? Or have your desires apparently been more important? Has your sexual desires compromised your sobriety? Use the below space to answer these questions and to journal ways could you improve your sexual integrity.

_____

_____

_____

_____

_____

_____

_____

_____

_____

_____

_____

_____

_____

_____

DAY SEVENTEEN

Word of the Day: *Joy*

Scripture: "Always be joyful. Never stop praying. Be thankful in all circumstances, for this is God's will for you who belong to Christ Jesus." (1 Thessalonians 5:16-18, NLT)

Quote: "I don't think of all the misery, but of the beauty that still remains." (Anne Frank, <u>The Diary of a Young Girl</u>)

Joy in the Midst of Trials and Tribulations

James 1:2: "Consider it pure joy, my brothers and sisters, whenever you face trials of many kinds...." (NIV).

Let's look at this word joy for a moment. Joy is defined as: Joy (verb): To experience great pleasure or delight: REJOICE.

To me (Phil), joy is not simply happiness. Happiness seems too momentarily fleeting. In the past, I felt happy when I had a good day at work or when the Vikings won, but eventually this happiness faded. Joy is much deeper and abiding.

Joy is different from happiness in that the word "happy" comes from the same root word as "happen": "hap." "Hap" means chance or fate. The feeling of happiness comes from what happens to a person by chance, but joy is a source of delight. This source of delight is what lies underneath all emotions, no matter what happens to a person. No matter what circumstances we are in, we can find joy.

So James here says to consider it pure joy, my brothers and sisters, whenever…whenever, what? Consider it pure joy, my brothers and sisters, whenever you face trials of many kinds. What? That can't be right? You want me to count it as pure joy during trials, during disappointment, during loss, during heartbreak, during death? What in the world is this man James talking about?

He's talking not about worldly temporal happiness which is dependent on our temporary circumstances, but rather spiritually enduring complete joy in the Lord. The Lord is sovereign over all things, including trials. In the midst of our brokenness, in the midst of our struggles, in the midst of the beautiful mess we call life, we can still find joy. We can still find joy in the midst of the trials, because pure joy comes from God--not from us--and is an enduring state of mind or attitude.

On November 15, 1989, I (Paul) was driving home from work, listening to a cassette tape on the Book of Psalms. I heard a passage that confused me, about men flying over our heads and God delivering us from the fire and from the water. Confused by those words, I made a left turn without looking for oncoming traffic and was hit at fifty miles per hour by another car head on. My car flipped entirely over high up in the air and landed on my roof. My car was totaled and the only part of it not collapsed was the part where I was hanging upside down from my seat belt. The other car was also totaled, but neither driver had a single scratch.

Someone called an ambulance when they saw me in my car, upside down, with fire and water spewing out of my deranged hood. But I sent the ambulance away since nobody was hurt, and a policeman pulled up just as the ambulance pulled away. The policeman saw me standing beside my car in my suit and thought I was a witness and asked me if the ambulance just carried away the body of the driver. I told him, "I am the body." He was surprised anyone could live through that. I foolishly climbed back through the window of my upside down car to get the cassette tape and my Dallas Cowboys Weekly magazine.

Later that night, I had a dream where Jesus told me to get the cassette tape and listen to the Psalms until I came upon a verse that would "hit me between the eyes." So I woke up and left the room so as to not bother my wife, and listened to the tape until I came to Psalm 90:12, where God said we should number our days, so we can walk wisely on the earth. I knew immediately what God was teaching me. I pretended like I died on November 15, 1989, and have considered every day since that day a gift from God.

From that day until today I pray a fourfold prayer every morning along with my other prayers. I pray that God will: 1. Help me to become more like him; 2. Help me to serve him; 3. Help me to resist sin; and 4. Help me to learn from anything that may go wrong that day—to have joy in my trials and tribulations because they serve a useful purpose—to help me grow to be more like Jesus.

By the way, the day after my accident, I called my godly mother-in-law to tell her about the accident. She was not surprised, to my astonishment. She said she had been praying every day that week that God would protect me if I had an accident. "Why would you pray something like that?" I asked her. She said that a week earlier, she had been reading Psalm 90:12, about counting our days on earth. That night she had a dream that one of her children (or their mates) would have a car accident soon, so she had been praying for our safety since that night. I told her about my own dream and my own experience with Psalm 90:12, only one verse out of ten thousand in the Bible. What are the odds that that was a coincidence? Probably one in a trillion or even less. That was an act of God, reassuring me that he meant business.

I (Phil) heard my kids singing a hymn the other day based on Psalm 118 and many of you might know this chorus. The hymn goes something like this… "This is the day, this is the day, this is the day that the Lord has made. That the Lord has made. I will rejoice, I will rejoice, and be glad in it and be glad in it." I never really understood the origins of the hymn. If you look at v. 22 – it says "the stone the builders rejected has become the cornerstone." This song is referring to Jesus and his death. Jesus is the cornerstone and he was being rejected to the cross. Now, the very next verse is about rejoicing about that day.

We are rejoicing about the day that Christ was crucified. We are called to rejoice in all things. Let's remember that no matter what happens to us, no matter what trials or tribulations we go through, we can always find joy in the Lord. We need to grab hold of God's pure joy. Choose joy, choose joy over resentments, choose joy over anger, choose joy over worry, choose joy over guilt and condemnation, choose joy over fear and anxiety, choose joy over worldly sorrow, choose joy over jealousy and envy. Accept the great gift today of the joy of the Lord. Make a decision today to choose joy.

Daily Surrender and Reflection

Please spend a few moments reflecting on the concept of joy. How can you choose joy today? Recovery is not without struggles, how can you intentionally find joy in Lord? Use the below space to answer these questions and to journal about how you could have a more complete and consistent joy.

_____

_____

_____

_____

_____

_____

_____

_____

_____

_____

_____

_____

_____

DAY EIGHTEEN

Word of the Day: *Idolatry*

Scripture: "No other gods, only me." (Exodus 20:3, Message)

Quote: "All addictions are idols and all idols are addictive." (Dr. Jared Pingleton)

Addiction and Idolatry

The following are the original twelve steps as published by Alcoholics Anonymous:

1. We admitted we were powerless over alcohol—that our lives had become unmanageable.
2. Came to believe that a Power greater than ourselves could restore us to sanity.
3. Made a decision to turn our will and our lives over to the care of <u>God</u> *as we understood Him.*
4. Made a searching and fearless moral inventory of ourselves.
5. Admitted to God, to ourselves, and to another human being the exact nature of our wrongs.
6. Were entirely ready to have God remove all these defects of <u>character</u>.
7. Humbly asked Him to remove our shortcomings.
8. Made a list of all persons we had harmed, and became willing to make <u>amends</u> to them all.

9. Made direct amends to such people wherever possible, except when to do so would injure them or others.

10. Continued to take personal inventory, and when we were wrong, promptly admitted it.

11. Sought through prayer and meditation to improve our conscious contact with God *as we understood Him*, praying only for knowledge of His will for us and the power to carry that out.

12. Having had a spiritual awakening as the result of these steps, we tried to carry this message to other alcoholics, and to practice these principles in all our affairs.

The term "idolatry" is an old-fashioned word which is seldom used in our fast-paced, modern, technologically-oriented society. When we think of an idol we generally think of an artistically carved, perhaps somewhat chubby little guy fashioned out of stone or wood whose head someone may rub for good luck as they walk by.

But our idols are typically much more subtle, sophisticated and serious than that. What is an idol? Simply put, an idol is something or someone we depend or rely upon instead of God. Idols are what we use to temporarily medicate our pain or turn to when we're hurting, and thus, can become something or someone we worship (consciously or not) instead of God.

Another way to understand idolatry is that an idol can be anything or anyone which comes in between us and God. In other words, the object of our idolatry can be something that isn't even necessarily even a bad or sinful thing, but something or someone we prioritize above our relationship with God. We can "worship" people, places or things above our relationship with God. But nothing or no one is worthy of that level of prominence or prioritization in our lives. We tend to serve and live for whom or what we worship, and only God is worthy of our highest devotion and our deepest love.

Ask yourself today; what are the idols I worship? To where, what or whom do you turn when you're hurting, lonely and sad? Many people become addicted to mood-altering chemicals, substances or prescription medications to soothe or try to escape from their pain. Other peoples' 'drugs of choice' are the relentless accumulation of materialistic possessions, gambling, sex/pornography, thrill-seeking activities, work, co-dependent relationships, sports, hobbies, entertainment, shopping, or the pursuit of fame and fortune.

So fill in the blank—what or whom comes between you and God? The success of our recovery depends upon how we acknowledge and address our "idols." As today's scripture teaches us, the first of the ten commandments God gave to Moses was to eliminate reliance upon anyone or anything else besides Himself.

When we cave in to the temptation to rely on a substitute or counterfeit for God in order to inappropriately attempt to cope with our pain and/or distress, we inadvertently start our slide down the slippery slope of addiction. Because all idols are artificial and illegitimate, not only do they not satisfy or meet our need, they deceptively promise more than they can deliver—leaving us subject to the law of diminishing returns.

Thus in addiction language, idols become habit forming because they involve what is called tolerance or habituation--that is they require progressively more of the same stimuli for the brain to derive the same physiological and/or emotional response. What used to work to medicate the pain gradually no longer does the trick. Thus our idolatrous "gods" progressively and deleteriously grab us by the throat-- insatiably requiring more and more until we end up becoming hooked.

In the Gospel of Luke, chapter 4 verse 8, Jesus addressed perhaps His greatest temptation from the adversary when He quoted from Deuteronomy 6:13 which declares: "It is written: 'Worship your Lord your God and serve Him only (NIV).'" He steadfastly refused to try to cope with His overwhelming stress and suffering by means of a shortcut or substitute. He kept His focus on the Father first and foremost.

These dynamics of the addictive process are encapsulated in the first three of the 12 Steps. We are powerless over our sin to the point that our lives become out of control and unmanageable. The Apostle Paul explained In Romans 8:15-20: "I do not understand what I do. For what I want to do I do not do, but what I hate I do. And if I do what I do not want to do, I agree that the law is good. As it is, it is no longer I myself who do it, but it is sin living in me. For I know that good itself does not dwell in me, that is, in my sinful nature. For I have the desire to do what is good, but I cannot carry it out. For I do not do the good I want to do, but the evil I do not want to do—this I keep on doing. Now if I do what I do not want to do, it is no longer I who do it, but it is sin living in me that does it" (NIV).

Therefore we must believe that God is greater than us. In Mark 10:51-52, Mark told us about a blind man whom Jesus asked: "What do you want me to do for you?" The blind man said, "Rabbi, I want to see." "Go," said Jesus, "your faith has healed you" (NIV). Immediately he received his sight and followed Jesus along the road.

As we decide to turn our will and life over to Him we trust that He can and will deliver us from our bondage. When Jesus called James and John to follow him, they believed Jesus, in faith, and followed him: "Going on from there, he saw two other brothers, James son of Zebedee and his brother John. They were in a boat with their father Zebedee, preparing their nets. Jesus called them, and immediately they left the boat and their father and followed him" (Matthew 4:21-22, NIV).

Steps 4-6 describe the dynamics of our sinfulness. From 1 John 1:8-9, we understand that "If we say we have no sin, we deceive ourselves, and the truth is not in us. If we confess our sins He is faithful and just and will forgive us our sins and cleanse us from all unrighteousness" (NIV). When we make a searching and fearless inventory of ourselves, admit our wrongs to God, ourselves and others and humble ourselves to ask God to change our defective character, we begin to become transformed.

The dynamics of this transformation are outlined specifically in Steps 7-9. The internal changes necessary for lasting externally manifested change and growth are profoundly articulated by the Apostle Paul in 2 Corinthians 7:10: "For Godly sorrow that is in accord with the will of God produces a repentance without regret, leading to salvation; but worldly sorrow (the hopeless sorrow of those who do not believe) produces death" (AMP). By asking God to remove our shortcomings, listing persons we have offended or injured and making amends, we will never be the same.

Finally, the dynamics of the ongoing recovery process are emphasized in Steps 10-12. A relatively obscure yet absolutely profound passage in the little letter of Titus (chapter 2, verses 11-14) offers positive, power-packed principles for our struggles with addictive idols. The Apostle Paul wisely counsels "… the grace of God that brings salvation has appeared to all men. It teaches us to say 'No' to ungodliness and worldly passions, and to live self-controlled, upright and godly lives in this present age, while we wait for the blessed hope---the glorious appearing of our great God and Savior, Jesus Christ who gave Himself for us to redeem us from all wickedness and to purify for Himself a people that are His very own, eager to do what is good" (NIV). Wow! What great news!

Through the powerful indwelling Spirit of Christ we can say no to our idols and yes to turning towards and living for God. This helps us exercise self-control over our controlling habits. Humbly admitting our brokenness, communicating with God and others about our wrongful attitudes and actions and then living in such a transparent and transformative way leads to freedom from our addictive idols. Consequently we can lead, mentor and disciple others with this great news, producing effective evangelism and marvelous ministry.

Daily Surrender and Reflection

Please spend a few moments reflecting on the concept of idols. What are the idols you worship? To where, what or whom do you turn when you're hurting, lonely and sad? It is good to have friends, sponsors and prayer partners to turn to when we are hurting, but are there any who have a greater place than God in our lives? So fill in the blank—what or whom comes between you and God? Use the below space to answer these questions and to journal about how you could lay down your idols and live more fully for God.

_____

_____

_____

_____

_____

_____

_____

_____

_____

_____

_____

_____

DAY NINETEEN

Word of the Day: *Feelings*

Scripture: "The heart is deceitful above all things, and desperately sick; who can understand it?" (Jeremiah 17:9, ESV)

Quote: "You cannot live life on what feels good. If we live our lives based on our desires, based on our feelings, we will lose our lives." (Pastor Phil Dvorak)

Just do the Next Right Thing

Matthew 16:24 Then Jesus said to his disciples, "Whoever wants to be my disciple must deny themselves and take up their cross and follow me" (NIV). Deny themselves. Whatchu talkin' bout Jesus? Our world is shouting to do what feels good, to listen to our hearts. Jesus you're turning this completely upside down. We must deny ourselves, deny our desires, our wills; we must put to death our old lives, and take up our crosses and follow him. Again, Jesus doesn't mince words here. He says anyone, who wants to be one of His followers, must deny themselves.

Those of us who have been in the rooms of recovery have probably heard statements like these; "feelings are fickle", "feelings aren't fact". You cannot live life on what feels good. If we live our lives based on our desires, based on our feelings, we will lose our lives. We must live our lives on what we know is right according to the word of God. It doesn't matter how wonderful it might feel. It doesn't matter how little the sin might seem, or what our culture might tell us. We must do what we know is right rather than what feels good. We must deny ourselves, pick up our crosses and follow our Lord to a new abundant life.

When my (Phil) first child Mabel was a newborn, we struggled. She was colic. Days on end she spent incessantly crying. Hours upon hours, we tried everything. It was about three days without sleep for my wife and at about three in the morning I got "the nudge." You know "the nudge." I had some choices. First, let me ask you, at three in the morning did I feel like walking upstairs and changing my daughter's diaper and sitting there with a screaming child? No of course not!

So I had a few choices. First choice, I could tell my wife "that's your job woman." I don't think that would have played out too well. Second, I could have lied to my wife. "OK honey, I've got this." Grab the baby monitor. Walk out of the room. Shut the baby monitor off and curl up on the sofa and go back to sleep. Third choice, I could walk upstairs, change my daughter's diaper, feed her, hold her, and rock her until eventually she fell asleep.

Let's look at these choices for a second. First choice, "Woman you should be barefoot, pregnant and in the kitchen; you take care of that child." How would that play out? Not good, correct? Second, the con game. I grab the baby monitor and act like I'm doing the right things. Sleeping on that sofa, sleep feels so good, but at some point I wake up and run upstairs to make sure I get there before my wife awoke. Walk into the room only to discover my daughter's diaper has blown out. She's covered, poop everywhere, I can see the bags under her eyes from crying all night long, and she now has a horrible rash. How do I feel in that moment? Like a piece of dirt. Like something you'd scrape off the bottom of your shoe. You see, if I did what felt good. If I went back to sleep and ignored the baby monitor, then I would end up feeling like a piece of dirt. Living life by our feelings won't result in a life worth living. Remember, the heart is deceitful above all things.

Let's look at the last scenario here. Three in the morning I get the nudge. "Ohhh, fine Hon." I walk up the stairs. I change her diaper, give her a bottle, hold her, rock her until finally she passes out, put her back in her crib and then climb back in my bed. How do I feel? Tired, exhausted, but fulfilled, a sense of accomplishment, joy, peace; tired, but good.

I did the opposite of my feelings. I did what I knew was right rather than what felt good and it ended with me feeling good. "Trust in the Lord with all your heart, and do not lean on your own understanding. In all your ways acknowledge him, and he will make straight your paths" (Proverbs 3:5-6, ESV). We need to do what we know is right rather than what feels good. No compromise...no middle ground. Like the Big Book says: "Half measures availed us nothing" AA p.64. Deny yourself and do the next right thing.

Proverbs 3:5-6 has been my (Paul) "life passage" since I memorized it at age 16. I think about that passage often as I make my daily decisions. A few years ago, I had a dream where Jesus was in the dream and told me to look up the Hebrew word for "acknowledge" in the Old Testament passage. So I woke up, got my Bible commentary, and looked it up. It means not only to do what God says to do, the right things, but it means to be aware that God is present in your everyday circumstances, thinking of you, guiding you, all in ways we cannot even imagine.

The next day, after that dream, I went to a Super Bowl party and put on an old pair of jeans. After the party, when I took off the jeans, a small piece of metal fell out of my pocket that I don't remember ever seeing before. I picked it up off the floor, and inscribed on it were the words, "In all your ways acknowledge him, and he will direct your paths."

It was affirmation from God that the dream had been from Him, and that He WAS AND IS present in my daily circumstances. I encourage you, right now, to look up that passage in your own Bible and write it down on a card or piece of paper and put it in your pocket and memorize it and live by it the best you can. You and I will make many mistakes in the years to come, but we will also avoid many by following this passage. Let the Holy Spirit direct you rather than your feelings.

Feelings are much misunderstood in our culture. Many people feel badly (translated "guilty") for feeling a certain emotion or not. But feelings are intrinsically neither good nor bad, right or wrong. It's what we do with them that makes the difference in our lives. Jesus experienced and expressed a huge assortment of feelings, but He never acted out His feelings in an immature, impulsive way. In fact, we know that "...we do not have a High Priest who is unable to empathize with our weaknesses, but we have one who has been tempted in every way, just as we are--yet He did not sin"

(Hebrews 4:15, NIV). Jesus felt every human emotion that we do. But He didn't His emotions control Him--He controlled them.

I (Jared) like to think of our God-given emotions this way: feelings are like a thermometer--they reflect the surrounding atmospheric conditions we are experiencing. Mature self-control and God-directed decisions are like a thermostat-- which exerts a moderating influence upon its direct environment. Are you more like a thermometer or a thermostat?

Another way to understand our feelings is that they can also function somewhat like warning lights on the dashboard of an automobile. Some people who grew up in dysfunctional homes where they were taught to ignore or deny their feelings are in danger of not being alerted to the fact that something is wrong inside and they need to attend to it. Sadly, many folks in effect try to just put duct tape over the light or reach down and jerk the wire to the dash. But that doesn't make the problem go away--it just gets worse. Warning signals, like pain, are a gift to a wise and mature person. They inform us that something is wrong and give us options.

To me both theologically and psychologically, the key to dealing with our emotions successfully boils down to this: do we let our feelings manage us or do we manage them? The way to tell whether or not this is the case for you is simple to identify. Here is what we need to remember: *healthy people talk out their feelings, whereas unhealthy people act out their feelings.*

Talking out our feelings is therapeutic. It is cathartic to talk out our feelings just as cleansing a wound, though painful, brings about healing. But to act out or act on our feelings just proves we are selfishly and immaturely not trusting in the Lord to direct our paths, which typically and tragically leads us into sin, symptoms and sickness.

Daily Surrender and Reflection

Please spend a few moments reflecting on your feelings. Have you ever been deceived by your feelings? In what ways can doing what feels good not end up being good? How can you know the difference between what feels good and what is good? Use the below space to answer these questions and to journal about how you could learn to deny yourself and do the next right thing.

_____

_____

_____

_____

_____

_____

_____

_____

_____

_____

_____

_____

_____

_____

DAY TWENTY

Word of the Day: *Redeemed*

Scripture: "Therefore, if anyone is in Christ, he is a new creation; old things have passed away; behold, all things have become new." (2 Corinthians 5:17, NKJV)

Quote: "Remember that you do not have to be perfect to have a relationship with Jesus." (Pastor Philip Dvorak)

A Beautiful Mess

Dancing With Judah

I (Phil) love my kids, but they are a mess. I have four of them and at one point we had three children three and under. It was insane. One day things had just gotten too wild for me at home. Everywhere I looked it was like a bomb went off. I knew that in order to escape I had to take at least one of the rug-rats with me. So, my two year old son Judah and I went on a field trip to Home Depot. I can now tell you from personal experience it's never a good Idea to bring a two year old to a hardware store.

Judah, my son, was the silliest little guy I have ever known. Like most kids his age, he just attracted chaos. He was a climber and a runner. So I kept rescuing my son from near death over and over again. He was potty training and I had to take him into the pit of hell, a public bathroom. So, I got down on his level and looked him in the eyes like I'm telling him the most important thing in the world. "Judah, remember you don't touch anything in the restroom. Absolutely nothing!" And with a little smirk, he would get these little mischievous smirks, and his little squeaky voice he said "yes Sir. I don't touch anything."

So we walked into the restroom and he was good for about two seconds. Then he began to start picking up toilet paper and all sorts of who knows what off of the floor. So I grabbed his little hands before he put them in his mouth, picked him up and washed his hands. Then I sat him back down and immediately he began to lick the sink. I lost it. So finally I got him in the stall, I covered the toilet seat with paper. My boy informed me "I'm a big boy now" and so he refused to sit down. So I attempted to have him stand on the rim of the toilet in order to get him positioned just right. He then started spraying everywhere, all over himself, the walls, my pants, everywhere.

After washing us both in the bathroom sink, we attempted to make our escape out of the store. My cart knocked a shelf and I turned around to see this gorgeous orchid and glass planter fly off the shelf. It hit the ground and broke into thousands of pieces. My son began to laugh, then he saw my face and the laugh was frozen mid laugh out of apparent fear of my reaction. Someone from the store came and started to clean it up. I headed again to the exit only to realize Judah had escaped yet again.

He was standing in the middle of the store with his hands in the air and he said to me, "Daddy will you dance with me?" Are you kidding, will I dance with you, are you crazy? Do you not see the chaos? Is there even music playing? My inadequacies began to creep in my head. Then I stopped, I heard the music for the first time, and in the middle of Home Depot I had one of the most spiritual experiences I have ever had in my life. I danced with my son. I looked like a fool, I smelled like urine, I can't dance, but I didn't care. My son was filled with more joy, more contentment in that moment than I would have ever believed. In the midst of the mess, I felt closer to God then I had in years. You see, I believe in a God who doesn't just call us out of darkness, but jumps right in, and jumps right into the midst of the beautiful mess we call life.

Think about this. I love the story of the birth of Jesus, because it is a beautiful mess. Mary was betrothed (engaged) to Joseph. I know engagement was a little different back then, but not that different. Picture this scene for a moment. It's an ultraconservative society and there is a teenager pregnant, not married, and the person she is engaged to isn't the father of her unborn child. In fact, she claims that God is the father of her child. When she goes into labor there is "no place for them in the inn." So she gives birth to Emmanuel (God with us) in a stable and lays the Christ child in a feeding trough (manger) as His bed. A room filled with animals and animal "stuff" is the birth place of God's son.

This is not the place you would predict a holy God to choose to have His son born. But that's why I love my God! My God is a God of redemption. He takes broken, messy, dirty situations and people and redeems them. He uses a teenage unmarried girl to give birth to His Son. He is born in the most humble manner possible. He spends most of his life working with His hands as a blue collar labor carpenter. Then he ministers to the outcasts, the brokenhearted, the sick, and the sinners of His day, only to die the death of a criminal on the cross. What a beautiful mess.

Jesus, the son of God, didn't come and live in a palace. He didn't demand to be revered as the God He is, but instead came to live in the humblest fashion possible. He surrounded himself with a ragtag group of not good-enoughs. A group of broken, messy, followers. Jesus didn't chose to change the world with armies, swords, legions of angels and lightning bolts. He will do that in the future, we believe, but not two thousand years ago.

Instead, He changed the world by rejecting fame, playing with children, living and eating with rejects, with the broken, and taking our sin, our brokenness dying on that cross for us. Jesus is attracted to losers, to the outcast. He spent time with has-beens, not good-enoughs, the hurting, and the sick. He came for you and for me. You don't have to have it all figured out. We just need to start. We just need to take his hand and let Him lead us towards the first bumbling, stumbling, teetering steps toward the spiritual life, even if we're not very good at it.

Romans 5:8 is one of the best and blest lines in the entire Bible: "But God clearly shows and proves His own love for us, by the fact that while we were yet sinners, Christ died for us" (AMP). When we were at our very worst is when He loved us the very best! Remember that you do not have to be perfect to have a relationship with Jesus. He died for us while we were in the midst of our sin. God was able to take one of the most horrific acts in all of history, the murder of His son, and change it into one of the most beautiful events in all of human history.

He took a murder and used it to show forgiveness. God loves you and wants to walk with you through this beautiful mess we call life. Recovery will be messy. However, God will help you find the beauty in the midst of the mess. If God can take a murder and make it the most beautiful event in all of history, think of what He can do with your life. God desires to take your mess and transform it into a beautiful inspiring message.

My son taught me a lesson that day. You see, in his adorable face with his arms outstretched, with his squeaky little voice, when he asked me to dance, standing in the middle of Home depot, I saw and heard Jesus in him. Jesus said "I came that they may have life and have it abundantly" (John 10:10, ESV).

The word redemption is a big fancy theological word which basically means the God delights in transforming blessings out of our brokenness. To redeem something means there is a clear recognition of something which was formerly deemed valuable, but for some reason there has been some doubt or disparagement cast upon that worth. The timeless and poignant story of the Prodigal Son illustrates that even though covered in pig slop (which would have been particularly offensive to an orthodox Jew), the Loving Father ran to him, hugged and kissed him, put a robe, sandals and ring on him and threw a big party. The son's worth was redeemed. That's a glorious picture of how our Loving Father feels about and treats each one of us when we come home to Him.

I think Jesus is reaching out his hands to each of us saying, "will you dance with me?" He says "I don't care that you smell like urine. I don't care what you've done, my heart broke when they hurt you like that, every time you stuck that needle in your arm, every time you put that bottle to your lips, I wept for you." "But in the midst of all this mess, will you stop, will you stop and hear the music, will you hear my still small voice, will you take my hand, will you let me hold you, will you dance with me?"

Before my mother died at the ripe old age of 97, I (Paul) had a dream about her dying and going to heaven. And in heaven, I could look up from earth and see her dancing with my father. I heard an entire four minute long song that I (having a musical background) wrote down and later published: "Dancing with Mother." In the dream and in the song, I yell up to my mom, "Can I come up there and dance with you and dad?" But she replied to me, "No, son, not yet. You will be here dancing with us soon enough. But remember the love you received from your family and from God, and go dance with the people of the world, spreading that love."

I woke up weeping, more from joy than from sorrow. Yes, God wants to dance with you. He wants you to experience His love and His presence. But addictions are caused by basically two things, shame and lack of connectedness. God wants to take away your shame. And he wants you and I to connect to Him and to significant others. We need each other to survive in this messy world.

Daily Surrender and Reflection

Please spend a few moments reflecting on this concept of redemption. Have you ever felt your life was just too messy and you needed to get your life cleaned up before you approached God? How can you approach God as you are and allow him to start to restore you? Can you see ways that God has begun to redeem your story? How might God use a sober you, to share a message of hope and redemption to others and "dance" with others? Use the space below to answer these questions and to journal your thoughts.

_____

_____

_____

_____

_____

_____

_____

_____

_____

_____

_____

_____

_____

DAY TWENTY-ONE

Word of the Day: *Serve*

Scripture: "But if you refuse to serve the Lord, then choose today whom you will serve...as for me and my family, we will serve the Lord." (Joshua 24:15, NLT)

Quote: "It is difficult to free fools from the chains they revere." (Voltaire)

Serving God by Letting Go of the Past

When we are in active addiction we know what it means to be enslaved but often we do not understand what it means to serve the Lord. The definition of serve: "to be a slave to, to be in bondage to, to obey, submit to, yield to, give one's self up to." When you serve the Lord, you gain so much more *from life than when you serve your addiction.*

Joshua 24.15 says, "But if you refuse to serve the Lord, then choose today whom you will serve...as for me and my family, we will serve the Lord." This verse urges us to make a decision, whom are we going to serve? At first, the notion of serving (obeying, submitting to, giving one's self over to) may not be appealing. We may even argue that we would never do so. However, Joshua makes it clear that, whether we like it or not, we are serving someone or something. Notice it does not say to choose whether or not we are going to serve; it says to choose whom we will serve.

In Matthew 6.24, Jesus expounds on this same theme. He says, "No one can serve two masters. For you will hate one and love the other; you will be devoted to one and despise the other..." (NLT). God asks us to serve Him, to give Him our all and to walk away from our past lives. He wants us to be fully devoted to Him. Some may think that He is asking too much. They say, "I love God, but I don't like the idea of having to give Him my all."

Costs of Serving an Addiction

That notion of not wanting to serve something or someone can be ironic, especially for the addict and alcoholic. After all, it is rare to find someone so intent on serving (according to the above definition) than the way us as addicts serve our drug of choice. We are willing to sacrifice everything for that next high, and the next, and the next and the serving goes on and on. Robbing family and strangers alike, stealing, lying—whatever our drug or drink demands, we willingly sacrifice in order to "gain" whatever it is that the drug will deliver.

What does the addict gain? That list is a long, depressing one: We gain broken relationships, failed marriages, lost jobs, legal issues (including jail and prison time), loss of health and this list goes on and on. SPEC scans measure the blood flow through all the various parts of the brain. I (Paul) have seen the scans of many people, including addicts. You can tell how much and how long a person has abused alcohol or other specific drugs by the pattern of brain damage and the size of the holes in the brain. Is an addiction really worth it?

Alcohol to excess kills liver cells, so when enough liver cells have died in a man, he can no longer get rid of the estrogen than flows in every man's veins along with mostly testosterone. Then the man gets the effects of too much estrogen, like red blotches all around the nose, impotence, and sometimes even growing breasts, called gynecomastia. Are addictions really worth it? Sounds like a great deal, doesn't it? In exchange for your all, addiction will wreak havoc on your life and will destroy you. This is dramatically reminiscent of John 10.10a which states: "The thief (the devil) comes only to steal and kill and destroy" (NIV). Joshua declares that he chooses to serve the Lord; decisions, just like the decision to serve addiction, always come with both costs and gains.

Gains from Serving the Lord

In Matthew 16.25-26, Jesus says, "If you give up your life for my sake, you will save it. And what do you benefit if you gain the whole world but lose your own soul? Is anything worth more than your soul?" (NLT). Jesus in that verse is explaining the costs and the gains of serving the Lord. First, what is the cost of serving—everything! We must be willing to forsake our old way of life, our sin, our selfishness, and our desire to serve our drug of choice.

As a result of serving the Lord and giving Him our very lives, we in turn gain our lives! In John 10.10b, Jesus makes us a promise about our lives when we choose to serve the Lord. In it, He says that unlike the thief who comes to destroy, He came to give us an abundant life, a life free from the bondage of addiction. He gives us a life marked with meaning and purpose, an abundant life that will continue throughout all of eternity. If we serve the Lord we will become more like Him—able to love and be loved more deeply. What in life is worth more than that? We even learn to love and respect ourselves more. The GREAT COMMANDMENT is to love God and others as ourselves. Choose today whom you will serve, your addiction or your God; as for me and my family, we will serve the Lord.

Daily Surrender and Reflection

Please spend a few moments reflecting on who or what you have served. How have you served your addiction? What has it cost you? What is keeping you from surrendering and serving God? What might you gain by choosing to serve God rather than your addiction? What are some practical ways you could start to serve God today?

_____

_____

_____

_____

_____

_____

_____

_____

_____

_____

_____

_____

_____

_____

DAY TWENTY-TWO

Word of the Day: *Submission*

Scripture: "My soul thirsts for God, for the living God. When can I go and meet with God?" (Psalm 42:2, NIV)

Quote: "The fact that we do not desire all of God, truly reveals that He does not have all of us." (Pastor Michael Eleveld)

Three Dollars Worth of God

I have the privilege of teaching a Seminary course on the Life and Ministry of Jesus. My class and I were reflecting on His three year public ministry. We discussed His rise in public popularity, followed by the crowds turning on Him, leading to His crucifixion. How could this happen? God on earth; the great "I AM" in human flesh. How could He not continually gain in popularity?

The truth is this: if Jesus was here with us today, He would face the same resistance to His ministry that He did back then. Why? Because we all have an ego-driven, self-absorbed desire to rule our lives and keep God at a distance. Jesus was gaining in popularity until He made it clear that He was calling His disciples to a radical surrender to God and His Kingdom. At that point, fringe followers began finding excuses to head home to the safety of a relationship with God that came with all the benefits and few demands.

We are guilty of the same thing, aren't we? We ought to be sold out to Christ. We ought to be all in with Him. Instead, we hold on to dark things in our lives and refuse to bring them to the only place they can be healed, the Cross. We want all the benefits of God and none of the requirements to follow Him of submission, servitude or surrender. I don't think that is going to help us, do you? Isn't step three all about surrender to God? "Made a decision to turn our will and our lives over to the care of God as we understood Him."

To surrender yourselves fully and freely to Him, to completely make Him your Lord (which means boss), means you have to "...have this same attitude in yourselves which was in Christ Jesus..." (Philippians 2:5, AMP) and humble yourselves in submission. You are no longer on the throne of your life; you yield your heart and your life (and your relationships and your dreams and your money and your stuff, etc.) to Jesus and submit to His guidance, direction and control. Do you trust Him fully and completely to obey Him and do what He wants?

The poet, Wilbur Reese, said it so well in his piece,

"Three Dollars Worth of God."

I would like to buy $3 worth of God, please.

Not enough to explode my soul or disturb my sleep,

but just enough to equal a cup of warm milk

or a snooze in the sunshine.

I don't want enough of God to make me love a black man

or pick beets with a migrant.

I want ecstasy, not transformation.

I want warmth of the womb, not a new birth.

I want a pound of the Eternal in a paper sack.

I would like to buy $3 worth of God, please.

This all boils down to one thing. The fact that we do not naturally or easily desire all of God truly reveals that He does not have all of us. God simply works with what we give Him. He will not violate our will. How can He fully restore our lives without us giving Him all of the pieces? When I give God all of me, then I will hunger and thirst for all of Him. Being "stingy" on step 3 does not protect me. Ultimately, it hurts me.

Romans 12:1-2, sums it up well: "Therefore, I urge you, brothers and sisters, in view of God's mercy, to offer your bodies as a living sacrifice, holy and pleasing to God—this is your true and proper worship. Do not conform to the pattern of this world, but be transformed by the renewing of your mind. Then you will be able to test and approve what God's will is—his good, pleasing and perfect will" (NIV). Submission is not a dirty word. It is the gateway to faith, fulfillment and freedom.

Daily Surrender and Reflection

Please spend a few moments reflecting on these concepts of submission and surrender. If you have worked step 3, have you been "stingy" with step 3? How could you more fully surrender your will and your live over to the care of God today? Use the below space to answer these questions and to journal about how you could more completely submit to and therefore be able to surrender to God.

_____

_____

_____

_____

_____

_____

_____

_____

_____

_____

_____

_____

DAY TWENTY-THREE

Words of the Day: *Self-Respect*

Scripture: "I can do all things through Christ who strengthens me." (Philippians 4:13, NKJV)

Quote: "No matter how you feel, get up, dress up, show up and never give up." (Regina Brett)

God Wants Us To Believe In Ourselves

I (Phil) returned home from work the other day completely drained. I was exhausted and filled with self-pity. My heart felt heavy due to a week of conflict and what I perceived to be countless failures. I had just enough energy to turn on my T.V., in hope of escaping my own thoughts. The week seemed to be filled with, as Solomon said, "chasing after the wind."

As I flipped through channels, for some reason, the fishing channel caught my interest. Standing on a boat was a surprising sight, a professional fisherman born without legs and only one partial arm. His name is Clay Dyer, and he is an extraordinary man.

This accomplished competitor has fished in hundreds of bass tournaments and won many. He coaches youth football (watching him catch a football is incredible) and he donates his free time by taking disabled children fishing. His friends can't seem to praise him enough. One friend says, "This guy gets it. Clay knows what life is all about, and he lives life to its fullest. Nobody ever got more out of life than Clay

Dyer." Clay explained how the other professional fishermen reacted to his disability when he started competing in tournaments.

"At first, the other fishermen were a little standoffish. They could not understand how someone who looked like me could fish, much less compete in a professional tournament. Most of the fishermen in my early days of competing were uncertain about my abilities – until they went on the water with me, saw me drive my boat and fish."

When he was born without legs and arms, the world would have had Clay believe he could not accomplish much. However, Clay was raised in a Christian family that made sure that faith was a strong priority. He has carried the faith of his upbringing into all that he does today, and he has never let his disability prevent him from believing in God and himself. He says Jesus Christ is his best friend and number one sponsor.

As I watched his story unfold on the TV, I saw the love of God flow from him to all who have been touched by his life. "I am really looking forward to seeing all the wonderful things that we can do to bring joy to those in need," Clay said. Through the television, Clay began to minister to me. My self-pity could not help but be lifted as I heard Clay quote Philippians 4:13, "I can do all things through Christ who strengthens me..." (NKJV).

What an amazing man! I turned the T.V. off and sat quietly reflecting. You see I have spent much of my life filled with self-doubt and insecurities. I struggle to believe in myself. As I sat there reflecting on Clay's amazing outlook, God spoke to me through Clay's story. "How arrogant, how arrogant" were the words I heard in my heart. I was confused. "Lord, I feel like a failure, like I'm worthless and you are calling me arrogant?" "Yes, how arrogant is it for you to not believe in yourself, when I believe in you?"

The Almighty God believes in you! He says you are worthy, because He is worthy. How prideful is it for us to think we know better than God about our worth. God certainly used Clay to humble me. Clay's story did not take away my struggles, but it reminded me of how much God believes in me.

God also asks that we believe in ourselves. Clay believes in himself not because he has great physical strength, skills, gifts, etc., but because he knows that God believes in him. "I knew I had a heart, a soul and a mind, which is what really makes a human being," Dyer says. "Anything else you have is a bonus." God bless Clay, and may his life continue to bless each person whom it touches!

Do you remember the GREAT COMMANDMENT?

Matthew 22:36-40, New International Version (NIV)

36 "Teacher, which is the greatest commandment in the Law?"

37 Jesus replied: "'Love the Lord your God with all your heart and with all your soul and with all your mind.' 38 This is the first and greatest commandment.39 And the second is like it: 'Love your neighbor as yourself.' 40 All the Law and the Prophets hang on these two commandments."

There are hundreds commandments in the Bible, but if you only remember this one, the Great Commandment, you will automatically obey all the others. All sins hurt someone. Learning to love God and others, as well as ourselves, keeps us from behaviors that hurt God, hurt others, or hurt ourselves. We have to fill our own love tanks before we have enough love to spill out unto others. This is totally different than the vain type of self-love—vanity that leads to sin. God wants us to have a healthy self-worth and a healthy kind of self-confidence. In fact, God says in Hebrews 10:35, "So do not throw away your confidence; it will be richly rewarded." (NIV).

Jabez was a godly man in the Old Testament who had the confidence to ask God to bless him even financially, to expand his territory. We could also apply the "Prayer of Jabez" to ask God to expand our beneficial influence to help others. The prayer is in I Chronicles 4:10 (NIV), 10 Jabez cried out to the God of Israel, "Oh, that you would bless me and enlarge my territory! Let your hand be with me, and keep me from harm so that I will be free from pain." And God granted his request.

Ask God today to bless you and keep His hand on you, and to keep you free from harming and causing pain to others or yourself. Psalm 139 tells us that God thinks about us, individually, so many times each day that we cannot even count them. With one arm, He holds us lovingly. With the other arm He leads and guides us. He created us in our mother's womb with the strengths and weaknesses we have.

What a beautiful picture of how important you and I are to God, in spite of our past failures. Let me ask you a question: What does God call someone who fails seven times in a row but keeps picking himself back up and, with God's help, keeps trying? The answer is that God calls that person a righteous individual. "For though the righteous fall seven times, they rise again" (Proverbs 24:16, NIV).

Daily Surrender and Reflection

Please spend a few moments reflecting on your self-worth and the fact that God believes in you. How do you value yourself? Are there things you are avoiding or not trying because of a lack of self-worth? Use the below space to answer these questions and to journal about what could change if you truly embraced the truth that your Creator loves and believes in you.

_____

_____

_____

_____

_____

_____

_____

_____

_____

_____

_____

_____

_____

_____

_____

_____

DAY TWENTY-FOUR

Word: *Character*

Verse: "Consider it a sheer gift my friends, when tests and challenges come at you from all sides. You know that under pressure, your faith-filled life is forced into the open and shows its true colors. So don't try to get out of anything prematurely. Let it do its work so you become mature and well-developed, not deficient in any way" (James 1:2-4, MSG).

Quote: "God is more concerned about cultivating Christ-like character in us than in creating creaturely comforts for us" (Dr. Jared Pingleton).

Cultivating Christ-like Character

It has been said that tough times never last but tough people do. Many times in life, and particularly in our struggles with recovery from our addictions, the times are tough indeed. Consequently, we may feel helpless, lonely, angry, confused, afraid, overwhelmed and/or hurt that God has not rescued us from the pain of these tough times.

Few of us ever want to go through what it takes for us to become tough and resilient. We know intuitively that the process of becoming tough is going to hurt, be hard and possibly horrible. Yet down deep, we also know that the pathway to truly becoming like Jesus—the toughest guy who ever lived—is often paved with things which are hurtful, hard or even horrible. Protective callouses on a worker's toughened hands never develop without first experiencing many painful blisters on tender skin.

As a kid, one of my (Jared's) biggest dreams was to play wide receiver for the Kansas City Chiefs. But due to suffering a severe back injury in college sports, my professional athletic aspirations ended abruptly. But I still love football, and even though I never made it onto the field in Arrowhead stadium as a player, as a Christian psychologist I have had the privilege of ministering to many of the players as a pre-game chapel speaker, and I have been friends with several guys on the team through the years who attended my home church in Kansas City.

Football is a tough, demanding (and for me a very fun and exciting) sport. It combines athletic prowess, precision teamwork, strategic competitiveness, mature self-discipline, focused concentration, brute strength, stamina and endurance. Due to some intensely painful experiences of abuse and abandonment I suffered as a child, I was already pretty tough mentally, emotionally and physically by the time I got to high school to play football.

Tom Landry was a godly man, and also the coach of the Dallas Cowboys during a twenty-year stretch of making the playoffs every year, including winning a couple Super Bowls. When a reporter asked Coach Landry how he had so much success with his men, he grinned and replied, "It's really quite easy. I just have to make a group of men do every day what they don't want to do so they can accomplish the dreams they have had since childhood." He was a godly man but a tough coach who got his men in better shape and more practiced than the other teams. He was kind and fatherly to his men, but demanding, to build their character and strength.

But unlike Tom Landry, my high school head football coach was just flat out mean. He was renowned for running the toughest practices in the state. Our first three days of camp every year consisted of three 3-hour practices per day in full gear for three days in the Midwestern mid-August 100 degree (or above) heat with humidity to match, without water—that was a "sign of weakness." It's a wonder no one died! Many of his methods are now illegal by the way. In between we lifted weights, did film study and tried to get five hours sleep each night on the gym floor.

Our coach weighed about 270 pounds and would often stand on our stomachs as we did leg lifts (I was 6' 2", 155 then—and believe me I kept my abs taut!). Hundreds of push-ups per day, dozens of 100 yard wind sprints, "Oklahoma" drills (full contact one-on-one head to head violent collisions), bear crawls the length of the field, blocking sled drills down the field and back and lots of reps for each play in the playbook were the norm for our practices.

But what our team all hated the worst was whenever our head coach was upset with us or thought even one of our 120 member squad was dragging or lagging behind, he would scream the dreaded words "to the hill men!" The "hill" was a steep 45 degree incline leading from the locker room to the practice field that was about 100 feet long. He would make us sprint up and back many times, depending on how hacked off he was.

What he then always bellowed after we were completely spent was "…builds character men; builds character!" Unfortunately I had to begrudgingly admit that in the fourth quarter in November, when the other team's tongues were hanging out, we were still fresh, focused and usually victorious.

So although I totally disagree with many of his principles, our coach nevertheless built a lot of toughness into us. And the Lord has used the fruit of the character and perseverance I painfully learned on that team many times since in my life. Those sore muscles, bumps, bruises, dings and minor injuries I played through taught me to keep going although my aching flesh screamed for relief and comfort as well as for me to quit. But you know what? Through the years I have persevered in many of life's toughest times from what I learned through the blood, sweat and tears I left on that practice field.

What I later came to learn about our "mean" coach was that he was bitterly disappointed when, after being drafted out of college by the Cleveland Browns, his knee got torn up in rookie training camp and he had to retire. Thus his dream of playing in the NFL nightmarishly died before it even began. So perhaps he unintentionally took some of that frustration, anguish and disappointment out on a bunch of high school kids.

He also did some specific personally hurtful things to me. I was one of only two Christians on the team (the other guy believe it or not is now also a Christian psychologist and felt persecuted by that coach for his faith as well!) and let's just note that he didn't seem to share or respect those same values. So needless to say, twenty-six years after my last high school game, I was astonished to run into my "mean" coach one weekend at a huge Promise Keepers rally (a huge Christian men's event of about 80,000)--ironically at Arrowhead stadium--the home of the Chiefs!

He remembered me, explained that he had just become a Christian a couple of years before, and even apologized to me for the hurts he had caused me. And most ironically, due in part to the character he had (albeit no doubt unintentionally) helped develop in me through those tough times, I had already forgiven him many years ago and we were able to share some wonderful experiences in our lives as Christian brothers!

Indeed tough times never last, although it may seem that way in the dark, lonely, excruciating moments of the adversities and sufferings we experience in life. But the truth is tough people really can and do last—and even thrive with the Lord's help! I certainly realize that high school football experiences are pretty trivial compared to what real life often has for us (plus I willingly subjected myself to those tough times in order to be able to get to wear that awesome and prestigious letter jacket which was unavailable any other way).

We all know that life's trials, trauma and tragedies are what are really "tough." These we do not choose. In those hurtful, hard and horrible circumstances we instinctively cry out in our anguish for comfort from our pain. We naturally desire relief and rescue, and as a result, are tempted to medicate our pain in inappropriate, addictive ways. It is precisely at these crucial points that our recovery process is either effected and energized or subverted and sabotaged. And the difference hinges squarely on our character.

In real life's crises, the eleventy-three zillion dollar question is, how can we allow the Lord to develop His character more fully in us? You see the deeper truth here is this: *character is not born in a crisis, character is revealed in a crisis.* Who and what and how we really are deep inside is made evident when we are in a painful test or circumstance.

Simply put, whenever we get knocked over in life, whatever spills out of us is what was already inside us. Jesus wisely observed that whatever is resident within our heart is what comes out of our mouth (Matthew 12:34). If we are wise, like good football players we prepare ourselves and practice ahead of time for the tests and unexpected situations life so often and unexpectedly throws at us. Jesus successfully handled His temptations and interactions with the adversary by the self-disciplined internalization of the Word of God (Matthew 4:1-11).

In Matthew 7:13-14, we read about the narrow and wide gates in life. Jesus challenged us to "Enter through the narrow gate. For wide is the gate and broad is the road that leads to destruction, and many enter through it. But small is the gate and narrow the road that leads to life, and only a few find it" (NIV).

So as we are traveling on our journeys down the narrow road to recovery, let's choose to draw closer to God. Allow Him to develop His character in us so that when we get blindsided and knocked down by life we turn to Him instead of to our false and counterfeit comforts which are so addictive and destructive. Even All-Pros get tackled. But the tougher they are the faster they get up. Therefore the question to ask ourselves is this: "Does this crisis reveal Christ-like character in me or my addictive cravings for comfort?" Our health and recovery squarely depend how we answer this crucial question. The tough things in life are good for us--they serve to help develop our character and thus become more like Christ.

Daily Surrender and Reflection

Please spend a few moments reflecting on your character. What are some crises you have encountered in your life? In what ways did these trials change you? How might turning to God during a crisis produce a different outcome than turning to the world's false, easy fixes? When a crisis comes, how can you choose to let Christ use it to build your character rather than letting it break you? Use the below space to answer these questions and meditate on these things.

_____

_____

_____

_____

_____

_____

_____

_____

_____

_____

_____

_____

_____

DAY TWENTY-FIVE

Word of the Day: *Struggles*

Scripture: "I have told you these things, so that in me you may have peace. In this world you will have trouble. But take heart! I have overcome the world." (John 16:33, NIV)

Quote: "The struggles of today develop the strengths of tomorrow." —Unknown

Bringing Your Troubles to God

So, you've started the journey of recovery and have begun the process of surrendering your will and the care of your life to God. As stated in Step Three, you've chosen to make a decision to turn your will and your life over to the care of God as you understand Him.

You're doing the right thing. You've got a sponsor, you're working the steps, going to church, and maintaining a conscious contact with God. As a result and at this point, you might expect things to be "smooth sailing." After all, you've surrendered your life to God who is all powerful, loving, and is a good God.

I mean, we expect problems while in active addiction, right? You have probably felt like you deserved those problems—that they were consequences of your actions, or possibly even that God was punishing you or at the very least, withholding blessings based upon your actions.

You are working on making amends, on doing the right things, and have changed your life for the better. One would think that from here forward it should be blue skies, the wind at your back, and blessings falling into your lap. That may be how you believe things should be, but in reality, you still are overwhelmed with problems.

But why? After all, you expected them when you were doing the wrong things. When that is not the case (which will often be true), we tend to think that we have done something wrong or that there is something wrong with us. "If only I would… then God would bless me and life would be wonderful."

God does want us to live an abundant and blessed life, but He doesn't promise we will experience heaven here on earth. He promises to help us on our journey through life here on earth. Heaven will be perfect and awesome, but that comes later. Everyone who Jesus ever healed 2000 years ago died of something later. Everyone you love will die someday. You will die someday, unless the rapture happens and you go up with the "uppertaker" before the undertaker comes.

The problem here is not that you are doing something wrong or even that you aren't doing enough right things; the problem is life happens. The problem is that we live in a fallen world that is far from perfect, in which we will have struggles and problems, regardless of how many things we are doing right.

In John 16.33a, Jesus says this about life on this earth, "Here on earth you will have many trials and sorrows" (NLT). Notice Jesus didn't say that those trials and sorrows would end once you turned your life over to Him, once you were doing the right things. He said the duration for those problems was "this life."

This may seem like bad news, and indeed, it does warn us that difficult times are ahead. In the end of that same scripture, Jesus says, "But take heart, because I have overcome the world." This is the same Jesus who in Matthew 11.28 says, "Come to me, all of you who are weary and carry heavy burdens, and I will give you rest" (NLT). When we are weary and feel overburdened, we can either pray for God to lift our burdens or pray for Him to strengthen our backs. In fact, it is probably a good idea to pray for both.

When God tells us in I Thessalonians 5:18, "In everything give thanks; for this is the will of God in Christ Jesus for you" (NKJV), He is telling us that we can be thankful even for the tough things that happen to us in life. The reason is that because, if our goal in life really is to become more like Jesus, rather than to experience heaven on earth, then the tough things in life are what help us the most to accomplish our goal of becoming more like Him. Martin Luther King is famously quoted as saying that whatever doesn't kill us makes us stronger!

When I (Paul), as a psychiatrist, ask any older and wiser person what was the time in their life when he or she experienced the most personal growth, nearly always the answer is during the toughest time in that person's life. Antiques are worth far more than brand new furniture, and antiques have nicks on them from all the experiences that piece of furniture went through in life. We have nicks on us too, but that just adds to our value.

Take heart, because Jesus has overcome the world. Jesus lived a life not free from struggles and problems. He overcame them and wants you to know that you will have struggles, problems and heartaches too. Jesus has been there, done that. In fact, "Because he himself suffered when he was tempted, he is able to help those who are being tempted" (Hebrews 2:18, NIV).

He understands, and He's here to help you in the midst of your struggles. Jesus is saying come to me—bring your troubles to me, and I will strengthen, comfort, and help you. The only one in history to have overcome this world is saying to you I have your back and will walk through these struggles with you.

Daily Surrender and Reflection

Please spend a few moments to think about some of the struggles you've been through. What has gotten you through these hard times? Next time tough times come, how can you give it to Jesus? Envision yourself laying your burdens (past or present) at the feet of Jesus. Use the below space to journal about your thoughts.

_____

_____

_____

_____

_____

_____

_____

_____

_____

_____

_____

_____

_____

_____

_____

DAY TWENTY-SIX

Words of the Day: *Free Will*

Scripture: "Live as people who are free, not using your freedom as a cover-up for evil, but living as servants of God." (1 Peter 2:16, ESV)

Quote: "Free will can be your greatest blessing or your worst nightmare. Which one is up to you." (Pastor James Exline)

The Blessing and Struggle of Free Will

"I'm an adult, and I'll do what I want." "No one is going to tell me what to do." How many times have you said either one of these statements? You might have gone to treatment, got therapy, you've been told what works and you know what you should do. However, there's just one problem— free will. Free will is defined as a voluntary choice or decision, the ability to act at one's own discretion. Free will is a gift from God. It is a blessing, and it can also be a curse. How we use it determines so much in life and in recovery. Deciding what we want, what we are willing to do and what we are not willing to do is all a part of free will.

The very first time we see free will as a potentially bad thing, or as a curse, is with Adam and Eve in the Garden of Eden. God creates man. Adam and Eve live in this paradise—no sickness, no physical or emotional pain, no addiction, no problems whatsoever. God had one rule, one restriction—don't eat from one tree. That's it, it was that simple. Use free will to obey God and live, use it to do what they wanted, their way, and live, but don't eat from that one tree. They decided what God said was not true, and that their way was better than God's way. Sounds familiar, doesn't it?

None of us would ever trust Christ as our Savior without the enablement of the Holy Spirit at that moment in our lives, but we still have free will. God wants to spend eternity in heaven with people who choose to accept Him. He knocks at the door of our hearts, and is not willing for anyone to perish, but still gives us free will. We are created in His image, and God has free will.

Very significantly, He chooses to never violate our freedoms He has given us and the wills He has given us. He is fully respectful of our individual freedoms and choices. Several examples of God's respect for our personal boundaries are detailed in scripture, including "Come now, let us reason together says the LORD…" (Isaiah 1:18, ESV), "Choose for yourselves this day whom you will serve…" (Joshua 24:15, AMP), and "… Now choose life, so that you and your children may live" Deuteronomy 30:19, NIV).

My (Phil) mother was diagnosed with diabetes several years ago. That was a life-changing, life-threatening diagnosis. Her life would never be the same, and free will would determine which way her life would go. She had two choices. She could use her free will to do the right things: change her diet, faithfully check her sugar levels, take the appropriate medicines, exercise and live. Or she could decide not to do any of those things, and get sicker and sicker, and possibly die.

She has her good days and bad days, but often she has chosen poorly. She loves her Coca Cola and her hidden stash of candy. She has used her free will, just like Adam and Eve, to do what she desired, what she felt like. You probably know the outcome. Fortunately, she hasn't passed away, but I fear without significant changes her health will start to rapidly deteriorate.

Those of us in recovery, like my mother, have also been diagnosed with a disease—addiction. It too is a life-changing and life-threatening disease. Just like Adam and Eve, just like my mother, we have free will, and how we use it will determine the outcome of our story as well. We have been told what works, what we need to do in order to stay sober and we have free will.

How are you going to use your free will? Will you do the right things— get a sponsor, work the steps, go to meetings, surrender to God and ask Him for His help in your fight against addiction? Will you choose to use this great gift of free will to help others and share God's love? Or, are you going to use your free will to decide that no one is going to tell you what to do?

Will you do what you want and decide what's best for you? Many of us, just like Adam and Eve, just like myself and my mother, have decided to use their free will to do exactly that. We do what we want, instead of obeying God's plan for our lives and doing what we know will help us stay sober and change this world for the better.

Free will can be your greatest blessing or your worst nightmare-- which one is up to you. The outcome of your story is still being written, and your free will is going to dictate the final copy. Use it wisely and live; use it poorly, and possibly die.

Daily Surrender and Reflection

Please spend a few moments and reflect on how you have used the gift of free will. What are some things you know you need to change, but haven't? What is holding you back from obeying God's plan for your life? Commit today to doing at least two things to help you in your journey of recovery. Journal those items here.

_____

_____

_____

_____

_____

_____

_____

_____

_____

_____

_____

_____

_____

_____

DAY TWENTY-SEVEN

Word of the Day: *Love*

Scripture: "The Lord your God is in your midst, a mighty one who will save; he will rejoice over you with gladness; he will quiet you by his love; he will exult over you with loud singing." (Zephaniah 3:17, ESV)

Quote: "Though our feelings come and go, God's love for us does not." (CS Lewis)

Does God Love Me?

"Does God love me?" seems like a simple question; one with the apparently obvious answer, "Yes, of course God loves me. He loves everyone." While we may know God loves us, how often do we feel or believe that God truly does love us? The most familiar verse in the Bible is probably John 3:16 (KJV), "For God so loved the world that he gave his only begotten Son, so that everyone who believeth in him should not perish, but have everlasting life."

He loves us enough to become a human in the form of Jesus, and to die on the cross for our sins. And, you know what? If you were the only person who ever lived, Jesus would still come to earth and die for you personally. Psalm 139 says He thinks about each one of us so many times each day we cannot even count them. He holds us with one hand and guides us through life with His other hand, giving us free will all along the way.

I (Paul) heard all my life the truth that God does indeed love me; however, it was several decades later when I truly believed and accepted the fact that God really loves me. Until then, God seemed like a distant, often angry God – the Almighty Smiter, if you will. This led to my vacillating between running from Him and attempting to be good enough for Him; neither of which ended well!

Paul's prayer for believers in 2 Thessalonians 3:5 is that the Lord would lead their hearts into a full understanding of the love of God. Again in Ephesians 3, his prayer is that they may "know this love that surpasses knowledge." This, I believe, is at the very heart of our relationship with God. We must come to know Him more and more, truly believing in and gaining a better understanding of His love--not merely intellectually, but also experientially.

I wrote a book in 2015 called "Experiencing God Outside the Box," in which I explained ten different ways that we get confused about what God is really like. One of them, for example, is whatever our earthly father was like. As a young child, learning to say your good-night prayers, you are thinking, "Dear Heavenly Version of my earthly father." If your father was absent, you will tend to think there is no God, or that He is off at a distance from you and not interested in you. If your father spoiled you, you will tend to get up in the morning and give God your list of things you want Him to do for you that day. You will tend to be a "name it—claim it" Christian. If he was abusive, you will tend to see God as abusive. Islamic terrorists think their God is calling them to kill everyone who does not see Him the same way they do, and follow the same rules.

Paul, who had a deep understanding of God's love, describes that love in Romans 8.38-39: "And I am convinced that nothing can ever separate us from God's love. Neither death nor life, neither angels nor demons, neither our fears for today nor our worries about tomorrow—not even the powers of hell can separate us from God's love. No power in the sky above or in the earth below—indeed, nothing in all creation will ever be able to separate us from the love of God that is revealed in Christ Jesus our Lord" (NLT).

One of the terms the Bible uses to describe God's love is the word everlasting. Everlasting is defined as: "undying, abiding, enduring, continual, persistent, uninterrupted." This means that it is without beginning or end; that which always has been and always will be. God can see into the future just as easily as He sees and remembers the past.

He didn't wait until you were born, or until He created you to love you. God knew you and loved you before you were born.

Did you catch that? God loved you before you could even try to be lovable! In fact, there never was a time when God did not know you and did not love you, and there never will be a time when He does not love you! God's love for you is not conditional on what you've done or what has been done to you. God loves you and "God showed his great love for us by sending Christ to die for us while we were still sinners." Romans 5:8 (NLT). *God cannot love you any more, or any less, than He does right now.*

My prayer for you is the same as The Apostle Paul's—may the Lord lead your hearts into a full understanding and expression of the love of God and the patient endurance that comes from Christ. Experiencing God's love in an intimate way will make you more able to genuinely love and be loved by others, and by yourself, disposing of your false guilt and shame.

The Apostle Paul powerfully prays for us to personally understand and internalize God's marvelous and magnificent love for us this way: "For this reason I kneel before the Father, from whom every family in heaven and on earth derives its name. I pray that out of His glorious riches He may strengthen you with power through His Spirit in your inner being, so that Christ may dwell in your hearts through faith. And I pray that you, being rooted and established in love, may have power, together with all the Lord's holy people, to grasp how wide and long and high and deep is the love of Christ, and to know this love that surpasses knowledge – that you may be filled to the measure of all the fullness of God" (Ephesians 3:14-19, NIV).

Daily Surrender and Reflection

Please spend a few moments reflecting on God's love for you. What might change if you truly embraced His everlasting love? Picture your Savior rejoicing over you and quieting your spirit with His boundless love. Nothing can ever separate you from His love. Use the below space to answer these questions and to meditate on these things.

_____

_____

_____

_____

_____

_____

_____

_____

_____

_____

_____

_____

_____

_____

_____

_____

DAY TWENTY-EIGHT

Word for the Day: *Forgiveness*

Verse: "For if you forgive others their trespasses, your Heavenly Father will also forgive you, but if you do not forgive others their trespasses, neither will your Father forgive your trespasses" (Matthew 6:14-15, ESV).

Quote: "Forgiveness is the hardest and most important thing there is."(Dr. Jared Pingleton)

Forgiveness is for Giving

Everyone experiences pain and suffering in life. Typically—and tragically—we receive our most traumatic wounds within the context of our closest interpersonal relationships. Herein lays a tremendous irony: we are usually hurt by and thus hurt those whom we love most deeply (Remember the old country music song which tells us we always hurt the ones we love?). As a result, the way we address and process these injuries holds enormous implications for our recovery. Our recovery absolutely depends on our giving the gift of forgiveness to those who have hurt us.

Forgiveness may be the most important *and* the most difficult thing in the world. After all, we gain eternal life by trusting Christ, thus getting forgiveness for our sins—past, present and future. In order to live a happy life, we must forgive others. If we hold bitterness in our hearts, we know from scientific research that we deplete serotonin from our brains, which causes us to become more and more depressed and anxious and develop insomnia and a host of other negative symptoms. When we forgive, our serotonin gradually gets back to a normal level in our brains. We need serotonin to experience love, joy and peace.

When we are hurt, our natural, reflexive inclination is to react in one of two ways (or maybe both). Either we take steps to protect ourselves from being vulnerable to further injury (by defensively withdrawing and putting up a barricade); or else we try to angrily lash back and inflict revenge on our offender.

But each of these instinctive reactions results in additional dysfunction, disharmony and destruction. Perhaps that's why Jesus confronted us so clearly in the Sermon on the Mount with the absolute necessity of forgiving (Matthew 6:14-15), and the Apostle Paul gave us a clear model on precisely how to give the undeserved gift of forgiveness (Ephesians 4:31-5:2). At times however, it may still seem or feel to be impossible to freely and fully forgive.

The truth is however, that whenever we do not forgive, we forfeit our personal power. Think about it this way: when we do not forgive, we unknowingly and unintentionally allow whoever offended us (whether it be some "jerk" who cut us off on the highway, or someone who truly— even deliberately—harmed us in some personally significant way) to distract and deter us from our normal focus in life. We automatically allow ourselves to become consumed with feelings and fantasies of retaliation and revenge. What we don't realize is this: *never does an offender control us more than when we do not forgive them!*

Wow, just let that sink in for a minute. So what are we to do? We were just driving down the road of life (perhaps for once!) minding our own business and now this selfish jerk has just messed up our whole day. We've all been harmed and it hurts like crazy. We want to get them back. It feels like we need to get them back! And yet to do so just hurts us, and them, even more. Down deep we all cry out that this is totally unfair!

Ok, so let's operationally define terms. Forgiveness simply means "giving up our right to hurt back." Yet to do so counteracts and flies in the face of the *lex talionis,* or "law of retribution," which is our universal human tendency and temptation to get someone back who hurt us.

That's why God has to tell us specifically not to take revenge (Leviticus 19:18, Romans 12:17-21). No one has to teach us to feel that we deserve "tit for tat." The ancient Code of Hammurabi taught an eye for an eye and a tooth for a tooth, which seems both reasonable and fair to our fleshly nature. However, God promises in Romans 12 to enact vengeance on those who sin against us, but in His time and in His own way. He will do it perfectly, even forgiving that person if he repents genuinely. When we get vengeance, we are foolishly trying to play God, thinking our way of doing so is better than trusting God to do it His way.

Unfortunately, when we act on this innate human impulse of revenge, we gain nothing and usually end up hurting ourselves as well as others. If I drive madly for nine miles, weaving through traffic in an attempt to cut off the guy who cut me off, I never get my 25 to 30 feet of pavement nine miles behind me back—I simply endanger the lives of my passengers and fellow travelers along the way. In the same manner, poking out someone's eye or tooth can't restore our own vision or smile—it just keeps ophthalmologists and dentists in business! Revenge is not only functionally pointless, it's counterproductive. It has been wisely observed that taking revenge is like drinking poison in hopes that our enemy will die.

Yet when we are wounded, our pain and suffering are real. To deny this, pretend it isn't there, or attempt to "spiritualize" it away is not only immature, it's unrealistic. Psychologically, we must grieve our losses in order to heal our hurts. And this work of grieving almost always is a multifaceted process, usually takes a long time and is a lot of hard personal work. We must labor our way through it in several stages over time, just as when we emotionally process a physical death. Without that Godly work, we will stay stuck in an immature and reactive state of mind, hell-bent on revenge. Otherwise, we will never move on to the mature and proactive stance of extending the gift of forgiveness to our offender.

Try this experiment: think of someone who has hurt you badly in the past. Now get an empty chair and put it in front of you. Imagine that the person who hurt you is sitting in the chair. Now look them in the eye, call them by name, and tell them how you really feel about what they have done. When you do this, your emotions will probably well up within you and you may even weep or get angry. Then pray for God to help you to forgive that person, not because that person deserves it—they probably don't. Forgive them with God's help so that you won't keep giving that person power in your life. Forgive him or her for your own sake and for

God's sake. You will probably feel greatly relieved, like a burden has been lifted off your back.

In the recovery process, steps eight and nine are often the hardest for many people. Healing the heartaches and hurts of our battered, bruised and broken relationships may feel overwhelming if not impossible. It may feel excruciatingly painful to face the shame, anger, fear, guilt and resentment of our past. To make ourselves vulnerable again by releasing others from the hooks and expectations of self-protection and/or revenge may seem ridiculous and ill-advised. And though we do need healthy boundaries and must guard our hearts (see Proverbs 4:23), giving up our right to hurt back and making amends when and where we can releases both us and our offender.

You see, forgiveness represents the very heart of the Gospel. The truth is that no one ever "deserves" to be forgiven. Not only is forgiveness unfair, it is also unjust. No one can earn or deserve it—much like all the other priceless treasures of Christianity, such as love, mercy and grace. That's why it has to be a gift which we freely give. No matter how deep the pain and disappointment you experience in life, remember this: *never are we more genuinely like God than when we freely give the gift of forgiveness to someone who doesn't deserve it.* This is how, who and what God is!

Forgiveness is the most expensive, essential and extravagant gift in the universe. It builds bridges instead of walls. It heals, transforms and redeems. We cannot fully and truly recover until we give, and thus receive from God, the priceless and precious gift of forgiveness.

Daily Surrender and Reflection

Please spend a few moments pondering if there are people in your life that may need your forgiveness. If forgiveness is the most expensive, essential and extravagant gift you can give, how could extending it to someone, though undeserved, change their life and yours? Can you remember a time in your life when unforgiveness had taken control of you? Ask God to help you to forgive.

_____

_____

_____

_____

_____

_____

_____

_____

_____

_____

_____

_____

_____

_____

DAY TWENTY-NINE

Words for the Day: *Spiritual Warfare*

Verse: "Put on the full armor of God, so that you can take your stand against the devil's schemes" (Ephesians 6:11, NIV).

Quote: "There are two equal and opposite errors into which our race can fall about the devils. One is to disbelieve in their existence. The other is to believe, and to feel an excessive and unhealthy interest in them" (C. S. Lewis, <u>The Screwtape Letters</u>).

Dastardly Dirty Deeds and Diabolic Deceptive Devices of the Devil

Newsflash: you have an enemy and he hates your guts! Whether we realize it or not, we are in a war. It is an unseen and unconventional war yet a very real and deadly war. But it's not a war you see video clips of on the nightly news or read about on the internet.

In <u>The Screwtape Letters</u>, by C.S. Lewis, the devil assigns demons to various people and instructs them how to manipulate the people to whom they are assigned. We believe in real demons and real angels. Probably all of us are sometimes manipulated and fooled by demons. Ephesians 1 describes the good angels as ministering spirits, sent to us individually to minister to us. We also believe we literally have guardian angels who probably follow us everywhere we go.

Several thousand years ago, Israel was ready to fight a battle in which they were greatly outnumbered. Elijah's servant was scared, and Elijah told him not to be afraid. Then Elijah enabled the servant to see the truth, and there were thousands upon thousands of angels on the battlefield, ready to defend Israel. Lots of people refuse to believe anything they cannot see. Yet we believe in the wind, even though we cannot see the wind, only its effects. But we would be wise to study what the Bible says about demons and angels and be aware of the spiritual warfare going on around us every day of our lives—just out of our normal sight.

The Bible tells us our fight is not against "flesh and blood" (Ephesians 6:12), but our battles are waged in the invisible spiritual realms, which are more real than our sensate experiences. And this spiritual warfare is very serious business. The Bible sternly warns us to "be alert and of sober mind. Your adversary the devil prowls around like a roaring lion, looking for someone to devour" (1 Peter 5:8, NIV).

That vivid imagery of a ravenous, roaring lion is absolutely terrifying. However, notice carefully that the text doesn't depict the devil *as* a roaring lion, but rather, *like* a roaring lion. The deceiver works by means of smoke and mirrors. The Bible promises that the real lion (King) of Judah will ultimately and completely conquer and triumph over evil and the evil one forever (Revelation 5:5). Furthermore, we are assured that "…when the enemy comes in like a flood, the Spirit of the LORD will lift up a standard against him" (Isaiah 59:19, NIV).

Meanwhile, back on planet earth in the here and now, we wrestle with good versus evil, light versus darkness and right versus wrong. These classic, timeless themes regarding the vicissitudes of human existence are the stuff of which countless books, poems, plays and films are made. And as C. S. Lewis wisely observed, some people err by dwelling on the devil and his dastardly dirty deeds obsessively while others attempt to deny and/ or ignore them altogether.

I certainly don't see Satan or his demons as lurking behind every bush or hiding under every rock as some do, but on the other hand, I don't conceptualize him as merely some antiquated abstract symbolic representation of evil as others do. Scripture teaches that he is a formidable foe and a ferocious force with which to reckon. Again, he is very real and he absolutely hates your guts.

But please bear in mind: your adversary hates you and is determined to destroy you--not so much for *who you are*, but because of *whose you are*. As any low-life, despicable, terrorist/bully/coward/intimidator knows, the most diabolically effective way to try to get at someone you want to hurt is to mess with their innocent kids. Satan hates and wants to hurt you because you are God's precious and priceless child, and he is jealous of Jesus because He is our virtuous and victorious older brother, called "the firstborn among many brethren."

What is important is to be alert, aware and advised of the adversary's strategies and evil mindset. In addition, it is crucial to note that although Satan is *opposite of* God, he is not *equal to* God. We are made confident and comforted in the truth that "…he who is in you is greater than he who is in the world" (1 John 4:4, NIV). There is an old country song that sings, "I've read the Book, and we win in the end!" The Book of Revelation tells even tells us how we win in the end. Nonetheless, we are commanded to not be outwitted by the devil's evil, cunning schemes (2 Corinthians 2:11) and to steadfastly stand for righteousness (Ephesians 6:10-18).

Given that he already knows he is an ultimately defeated foe and has limited time and resources, Satan is totally hell-bent on hurting God as much as he can as long as he can by hurting God's children (us) as much as he can. I must unfortunately and begrudgingly admit that I do admire his work ethic: he is determinedly dedicated to delivering deception, death and destruction, stays fully and fiercely focused and doesn't seem to take a lot of sick leave or vacation time! Accordingly, it seems wise for us to familiarize ourselves with his schemes and understand them so we can avoid falling into his traps (1Timothy 3:7). Addictions are just one of many potential traps set by the adversary.

From a careful clinical consideration of both God's Word and of His people, I (Jared) believe we can observe a pronounced and purposeful pattern of battle strategies the evil one utilizes to attempt to harm us. We need to learn to recognize what those strategies are so that we can resist the devil to cause him to flee from us (James 4:7). Try to identify which of the following demonically-orchestrated, progressively intensifying battle plans and spiritual warfare tactics the enemy of your soul uses to hurt you:

- **Distract:** Many times the simplest way to effectively neutralize an enemy is to simply keep them preoccupied with something or someone else. It seems this is the adversary's most common weapon, and it saves him from having to use his limited munitions supply of larger artillery. For example, any ordinary addiction ostensibly functions to keep our mind off our pain yet it also keeps our focus on ourselves instead of God and His plan, program and purpose for our lives. Whenever our attention is diverted from our goal, often our energies are as well. Life has many natural, built-in things—many of which are intrinsically good--which can easily distract us from our assignments in the spiritual battles we are called to fight (caring for spouses, children, extended family, work, busyness, hobbies, etc.). Thus we are called to fix our eyes on Jesus (Hebrews 12:1-2) so we can avoid the easily entangled elements of sin.

- **Divert:** After we are distracted it is fairly easy to get us off track from pursuing and attaining our goals of living a righteous life. A commonly used military strategy is to create a diversion. After our attention is effectively diverted, the focus of our energies can effectively be deterred so we are not locked in on our targets and/or we can be tempted to drop our guard. If a bullet or missile is only a few degrees off, it will likely miss its intended target, rendering it ineffectual. At best, when we are forced to take a detour in life, we are inconvenienced and delayed. Sometimes all it takes for a martial arts combatant or offensive lineman in football to win is to slightly redirect the opponent's energies and efforts, thus successfully negating them. Again, it saves our enemy bullets when he can merely get us off track from accomplishing God's will. He can 'win' without firing a shot.

- **Discourage:** Keep in mind our adversary is exceptionally evil and patiently persistent. But he doesn't just want to win the battles; he want wants to ultimately win the war. The way he does that with many Christ-followers is to sideline them with a spirit of discouragement. When we are beaten, battered, bloodied and bruised, it's natural to want to go back behind the front lines to lick our wounds. And when we suffer "friendly fire" or get shot in the back by fellow Christian soldiers, it's understandable that we feel bad, bummed, betrayed and bitter. War hurts. Battles are scary. Injuries take time to heal. We get exhausted. And we commonly experience Post-Traumatic Stress Disorder from our battle scars, which results in our feeling downtrodden, depleted, dejected and depressed.

- **Defeat:** However, our enemy is not content with just taking us out of the battle emotionally. He wants to trounce us soundly, to demoralize us and to utterly defeat us. He keeps score. He brings up the past and functions as a tour guide for our guilt trips. He is even known as the Accuser (Revelation 12:10) of the brothers, trying to always make us feel, act and end up defeated. We must remind ourselves that there is no condemnation to those who are in Christ (John 3:17; Romans 8:1-2) and that even in death, He provides us with the victory (1 Corinthians 15:54-58; 1 John 5:4). We are not the ones who are losers, our adversary is (Psalm 60:12). If you had critical parents when you were growing up, you may go through life continuing to be self-critical, even after moving away from the critical parents. You are doing the work of demons on yourself. Satan may not need to assign any demons to you if you are doing a good enough job of demonizing (accusing) yourself, since that is the job of demons. So, right this very moment, take a brief break and get your Bible. Now open to a blank page in the back of it, and put down today's date, and a pledge to yourself to not say anything negative to yourself that you would not say to your best friend under the same circumstances. Then sign this pledge, realizing you won't be perfect at doing this either. We ask you to do this because you would certainly tell your best friend the truth, even if you lie to yourself by being overly self-critical, creating false guilt.
- **Devour:** What is it that eats you up? Or eats away at you? Is it an addictive substance or behavior? Do painful memories or old hurts and fears gnaw at you? What negative or harmful thoughts consume you? Do you frequently swallow hurtful emotions? These are often the heavy artillery that the enemy of your soul launches at you. These missile strikes are designed not only to immobilize you but to take you out. And as earlier noted, the adversary--like any cowardly predator--is slyly sneaking and slinking around looking

for a vulnerable, wounded, frail, sickly, damaged member of God's flock to launch a surprise attack upon and chew up (1 Peter 5:8).

- **Destroy:** Finally, the devil isn't content to only distract, deter, discourage, defeat and devour you. John 10:10 gives an insightful job description of his motive, methods and mission: he comes to steal, *kill and destroy* (emphasis added). Please get this clearly: his devilish design is to totally and completely annihilate you. He is relentless, ruthless and reprehensible. Jesus defined him as a liar and a murderer—that is who and what and how he is (John 8:44).

So don't let yourself feel helpless, overwhelmed and victimized. Put on the full armor, assume your position and take your stand in the battle and wage war against what is destroying you. Instead of succumbing to the evil one and becoming a casualty, choose to live out each day the principles of life Jesus has fought so hard for on our behalf. Recovery is a process. Remember, Jesus came that we may have life—abundantly or to the full (John 10:10). And best of all: we are overcomers as a result of Jesus' sacrifice for us and by sharing our story or testimony (Revelation 12:10-11). So take your stand, you are victorious!

Daily Surrender and Reflection

Now take a few minutes to think of ways Satan and his demons have tricked you in the past, or are tricking you in the present, or might plan to trick you in the future. Think of lies you tell yourself, especially negative lies you tell to yourself, and list these. And be sure to write down that pledge to yourself to do the best you can to tell yourself the truth in the future, like you would your best friend. In fact, pledge to become your own best friend.

_____

_____

_____

_____

_____

_____

_____

_____

_____

_____

_____

_____

_____

DAY THIRTY

Word: *Heart*

Verse: "Above all else guard your heart, for everything you do flows from it" (Proverbs 4:23, NIV).

Quote: "Will you allow the hurts in your life make you bitter or better?" (Dr. Jared Pingleton)

How to Guard Your Heart

Today's verse is a fascinating one. Consider the first three words...it says *nothing is more important* than to guard our hearts! Yet who teaches us to do so? Or how to do it? What is it that we are to guard against? What does that really mean or look like? And what is meant by 'heart?'

The Hebrew and Greek words translated as "heart" occur nearly 1000 times in the Bible. So clearly this concept is extremely important to God, and hence to us. What scripture is referring to by 'heart' is not the fist-sized pump in our chest, but rather, the affective center of our being—our inner personhood, moral character and core identity. This is the term used by Jesus when He differentially diagnosed good people from evil ones. He explained "The good person out of the good treasure of his heart produces good, and the evil person out of his evil treasure produces evil, for out of the abundance of the heart his mouth speaks" (Luke 6:45, ESV).

Simply put, whenever we get unexpectedly knocked over in life, whatever is inside us is what spills out. When we get cut off on the freeway by some jerk, what is our immediate reaction? I'll tell you what it is—it's whatever the overflow of our heart is. And what flows out is what we put in it or permit to enter into it. That's why we need to so strongly guard our hearts.

The original Hebrew word picture in today's text is both dire and dramatic: it depicts a super tough, fully armored warrior trained for battle (think Navy SEAL/Delta Force/Army Ranger type of elite soldier) who is garrisoned to protect all of our water supply. Nothing or no one is getting by without his permission.

Today, we pretty much take for granted easily available access to pure sources of hydration. But if you lived 3000 years ago in the desert you would be acutely aware of whether or not you could rapidly, regularly and reliably obtain clean drinking water. If your enemy poisoned, polluted or purloined your water supply, your chances of survival would be bleak indeed. You would die very soon.

So when you reread the above verse, consider the absolute life and death intensity of this scenario. After oxygen, our bodies require water for survival more than anything else. In the same way, our spiritual and psychological lives absolutely depend on us guarding our heart with all our might and with all the fight within us. Scripture teaches we must guard our heart in several key areas:

- **Hurts:** Everyone experiences pain and suffering in life; the challenge is how we get appropriate care for our wounds. If a physical wound is not cleansed and treated (which often hurts more than the original injury itself) we realize we run the risk of infection. The same is true with our emotional and relational injuries: traumas, trials and tragedies can all continue to hurt us, even disable us, if left untreated. Attempting to ignore or deny our hurts can seem like toughness, even heroism at first, but then we are ironically more vulnerable to reinjury and ultimately even disability. We must let God heal our hurting hearts as King David cried out to Him: "For I am suffering and needy, and my heart is wounded within me" (Psalm 109:22, AMP). Yet we have confidence that "The Lord is close to the brokenhearted and saves those crushed in spirit," and likewise can take comfort that "He heals the brokenhearted and binds up their wounds" (Psalm 34:18; 147:3, NIV).

- **Hungers:** Our human appetites are longings which are normal, natural and necessary. Yet when we obsess about or are controlled by them, we can be destroyed by them. For example, we all long for and need acceptance, attachment, attention, approval, affection, appreciation and affirmation. But when we are empty of these good things, we can be tempted to fill these needs with cheap substitutes with which the enemy of our souls wants to destroy us. Pursuing our fleshly appetites can certainly lead us astray, which is why we must guard our hearts and look to the Lord to nurture and sustain us. David's prayer for us was "May He grant you your heart's desire and fulfill all you plans" (Psalm 20:4, AMP) as he also encouraged us to "Delight yourself in the LORD, and He will give you the desires of your heart" (Psalm 37:4, ESV). Instead of allowing our appetites to be addictive, we should "…give thanks to the LORD for his unfailing love and his wonderful deeds for mankind, for He satisfies the thirsty and fills the hungry with good things" (Psalm 107:8-9, NIV). God made our hungers; His 'cooking' is both filling and nutritious! Ask yourself today: "for what am I hungry?" Then take what's eating at you to God in prayer.

- **Habits:** Habits are neither intrinsically good or bad—it's whether we control them or they control us. Besides obvious addictive behaviors, most people have many other harmful habits of which they may not even be consciously aware. Some of the most common ones are: gossiping, laziness, self-centered attitudes and actions, judging others, wasting time, disrespectfulness, negative thinking, greediness and apathy. Proverbs 20:9 points out how all of us are subject to sinful habits, asking rhetorically "Who can say, 'I have kept my heart pure; I am clean and without sin?'" (NIV). We must cultivate habits of spiritual disciplines as did King David who famously said: "Your word I have treasured and stored in my heart, that I may not sin against You" (Psalm 119:11, AMP). According to Stephen Covey, it only takes a month to change or establish a habit. If you will study verses 30-36 of Psalm

119, David demonstrates how he determined to habitually study, follow and obey God's laws/commands/statutes/decrees and turn his heart to God.

- **Humiliations:** It may very well be that nothing hurts psychologically more than the toxic emotion of shame. From Genesis 3 on, shame has been the bane of human existence. Shame and lack of connectedness are considered the two primary causes of most addictions. The classical hallmark of a dysfunctional family system is shaming and controlling behavior by means of humiliation and ridicule. Shame causes us to instinctively hide and pull in instead of confidently reaching out to know and be known—which is God's pattern and purpose for relationship. Shame causes us to be fearful, to experience diminished self-esteem, become withdrawn and inhibited and in extreme cases, become absolutely paralyzed to the point of becoming disabled and nonfunctional. Kind David was very familiar with the devastating effects of shame, mentioning it over forty times throughout the Psalms. In Psalm 25:2-3 he implores God to not let him be put to shame because he has trusted in God. Psalm 34:5 assures us that "Those who look to Him are radiant; their faces are never covered with shame" (NIV). And in Psalm 119, he links obedience to God's commands with never having to experience shame (verses 6, 31, 46, 78, 80). Obedience to our Lord is obviously the best way to guard our heart from humiliation.

- **Horrors:** Terror, trauma and tragedy certainly harm our hearts. The deleterious and destructive effects of horror define and delineate the nature of Post-Traumatic Stress Disorder and can last for generations. When we experience our world as being fundamentally unsafe, we generally react with one of the following: fight, flight or freeze. The overwhelming sense of powerlessness, fear and helplessness can cause us to lash out, blindly try to escape, or just shut down. While we can certainly guard our hearts from some horrifying experiences (e.g., garbage movies, violent video games, other sinful 'entertainment,' etc.), sometimes life throws things our way that can harm us horribly. Here the Apostle Paul tells us to "Let the peace of Christ [the inner calm of one who walks daily with Him] be the controlling factor in your hearts [deciding and settling questions that arise]. To this peace indeed you were called as members in one body [of believers]. And be thankful [to God always]" (Colossians 3:15, AMP). Mature 'heart-guarders' "...will have no fear of bad news; their hearts are steadfast, trusting in the LORD. Their hearts are secure, they will have no fear..." (Psalm 112:7-8, NIV). Finally, the ongoing, progressively developed self-discipline of always thinking about the good things in life (Philippians 4:8) results in the peace of God which guards our hearts and minds (Philippians 4:7).

- **Hatreds:** We rarely hate someone immediately. Usually hatreds are harbored in our hearts over long periods of time, incubating from old heart pain we have not dealt with. The process of hating another person or oneself usually results from unforgiven slights, snubs, sarcasms, slurs and sufferings. We feel victimized and therefore vindictive and vengeful. When we allow hatred to take root in our heart, it tends to accumulate and escalate into destructive dynamics such as prejudice, judgementality, arrogance and holding grudges. Resentments result in retaliation and retribution. The Old Covenant sternly warns us "Don't secretly hate your neighbor. If you have something against him, get it out in the open..." (Leviticus 19:17, MSG). Hatred will eat us, and others, up. As for self-hatred, the Apostle John gently consoles us that God is greater than our hearts whenever our heart condemns us (1 John 3:19-20), so because we have been forgiven, we can forgive ourselves and others. When we allow ourselves to be consumed by feelings of hatred, we allow the hated person to control us instead of God.

- **Hardnesses:** Of all the things from which we must guard our hearts, perhaps the most serious and significant is to guard against it becoming hardened. Like hatred, hard-heartedness is also typically a gradual degenerative process. When we lose our pliability we can no longer be easily shaped and molded. When we lose our flexibility we can no longer stretch or bend, we break. And when we lose our softness, we become insensitive, brittle and cold. When we harden our heart, we become incapable of loving or being loved; in fact, Jesus cited this as the rationale to concede allowing divorce in adulterous marriages (Matthew 19:8-9). The Bible specifically warns us to not allow ourselves to become hard-hearted to our siblings (Deuteronomy 15:7) and the poor (Proverbs 29:7), but mostly not to allow ourselves to become hard-hearted toward God (2 Chronicles 36:13, Hebrews 3:8).

There are over seven billion people on planet earth, and to some extent or another, all of us feels somewhat like a "nobody." Thus, our natural tendency is to go through life in a foolish rat race, trying to prove to others and ourselves that we are not a nobody. We do this primarily through sex, power and money, but also in other ways. Our hearts are both deceitful and deceived. The Prophet Jeremiah said (In Jeremiah 17:9; KJV), "The heart is deceitful above all things, and desperately wicked. Who can know it?" Just think about that for a moment. The most deceitful thing in God's universe is the human heart—including mine and yours. And who can comprehend the extent of it? Probably none of us. But we can choose to not believe the lies and accept the fact that, in Christ, we are a somebody. We are a child of the living God, with eternal life. Believe the truth with your clean heart and commit your life to Christ, to serve Him and to learn to love and be loved like He loves and is loved.

So more important than anything else in your life, guard your heart. We all get beaten, bloodied, battered and bruised in life. And those wounds definitely hurt. The question is, will you allow those hurts to make you bitter or better?

Daily Surrender and Reflection

Now take a few minutes to list ways that your own heart has been deceived. List some ways you have foolishly experienced the rat race of life. List some things you can do about it and substitute in its place. List some of the hurts, hungers, habits, humiliations, horrors, hatreds and hardnesses you have experience in life and ways you can heal from these and get past them.

_____

_____

_____

_____

_____

_____

_____

_____

_____

_____

_____

_____

_____

_____

_____

ABOUT THE AUTHORS

Pastor Philip Dvorak

Pastor Phil Dvorak is the founder and president of the Recovery Church Movement. Recovery Church Movement (RCM) is a growing network of Recovery Churches reaching and training those in early recovery to grow in their faith and recovery. He has served as a pastor, church planter, licensed mental health clinician, and ministry executive. However, his passion for those impacted by addiction is palpable.

Phil has personally worked with thousands of individuals. He is ordained by the Christian & Missionary Alliance and is a licensed mental health counselor. His treatment curriculums have been published and implemented by multiple treatment centers across the country.

He has a passion for seeing people recover from the disease of addiction and be a part of the solution to this crisis in our nation. He is a devoted husband, father, and servant leader. Phil and his wife Sara have five children. "Pastor Phil Dvorak is fast becoming one of the foremost leaders in the field of Christian addiction treatment. His compassionate, insightful, yet firm approach connects to your heart in a truly life-giving way" - Dr. Tim Clinton, President of the American Association of Christian Counselors.

Dr. Paul Meier

Paul Meier, MD, is considered by many to be a founding father of the Christian psychology movement. He is the founder and president of the non-profit, national chain of Meier Psychiatric and Christian Counseling Clinics consisting of twelve locations across seven states.

He hosted a national daily live broadcast on 400 stations to an average of two million people a day for over twenty years. Dr. Meier was also given the opportunity to spread Christian psychology by writing over 100 published books that have sold well over 8 million copies in 30 languages. He has discussed his books on many Christian and secular TV and radio programs. Dr. Meier also does a monthly secular podcast, *Mental Health News Radio*, to 171 nations.

Dr. Meier has travelled throughout the world on mission trips to train pastors, missionaries, lay counselors, professional counselors, and many others about how to integrate the Bible with up-to-date psychological research and medications to treat psychiatric illnesses. "Christian psychology" and "Christian psychiatry" are helpful tools to reach people around the world who would normally not come to churches or pastors for help. He has spread Christian psychology in unexpected countries like Russia, Israel, and Cuba and throughout Europe and South America. Dr. Meier continues to see psychiatric patients and administrate his national chain of non-profit Meier Clinics, with more information available at: www.meierclinics.com.

Dr. Jared Pingleton

Dr. Jared Pingleton is a Christ-follower, husband, father, and grandfather. He is also a third-generation minister, clinical and consulting psychologist, professor, author, and speaker who is passionate about communicating Jesus' love, mercy, and grace to a hurting and conflicted world. A respected leader in the Christian mental health field, Jared has been in professional practice since 1977 offering help, hope, and healing to thousands of individuals, couples, families, and churches.

Dually trained in theology and psychology, he has been a professor at several Christian universities and seminaries and served on the pastoral staff of two large churches where he founded and directed church-based community counseling centers. *He has authored, co-authored or edited ten books, including: The Care and Counsel Bible, Mental Health Ministry in the Church, The Struggle is Real: How to Care for Mental and Relational Health Needs in the Church, and Making Magnificent Marriages.*

Dr. Pingleton has also served in various leadership positions at the American Association of Christian Counselors, as Director of Counseling Services at Focus on the Family, and currently maintains a private practice.

Dr. Pingleton has extensive national and international media experience--appearing as a guest, host, or co-host on hundreds of television and radio programs and in many leading print publications. He maintains several professional affiliations, and is a popular national and international speaker and conference leader. For more information about him and his resources visit: www.drpingleton.com.